Contents

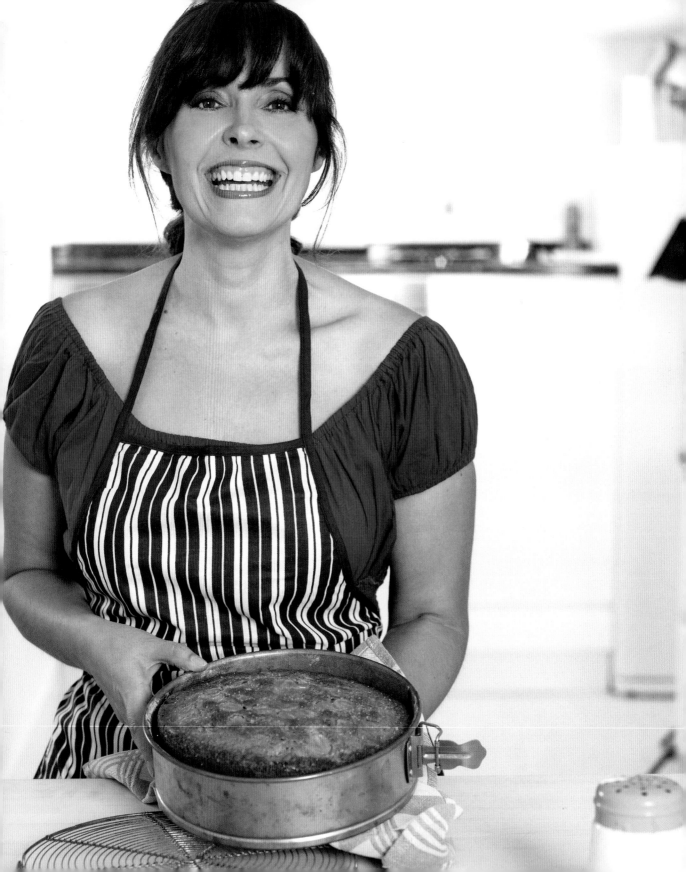

introduction

Life is too short and time is too precious not to make the most of a heavenly pud! When I thought about writing *Have Your Cake And Eat It Too* it was a very easy decision to make. You see, although healthy eating for me is a more than a lifestyle choice – it's actually a life or death choice – I also appreciate how important treats are. Food has to do many jobs for us. It has to satisfy our hunger and it has to give us essential nutrition to help us stay fit, well and strong. But food also needs, sometimes, to support us emotionally. When we are a little low and down in the dumps, a bit of sugar can boost the endorphins and give us a lift. A great meal with friends and family is a treat and shows a kinship; and as food is the glue that holds us all together, finishing a delicious meal off with a heavenly dessert makes us all feel satisfied and worthy of the treat before us.

Having said all that, and keeping in mind our need to stay fit and well, I am always mindful that to enjoy our greatest pleasures guilt-free, sometimes a little tweaking of old favourite recipes is necessary!

In this book I hope I have offered you some perfect, healthier alternatives to some old-fashioned classics and some new ideas to try too. In some of my recipes you will notice that I've managed to lose the fat all together; in others I have cut the fat content in half by lessening the quantity or using a low-fat ingredient. In all the recipes, I have followed my general rule of adding as much benefit, nutrition and flavour to my dish as possible. So even though a particular dish may have some fat content, it will be balanced by added nutrition to boost your health. Remember, these aren't dishes to serve up everyday but they will help you balance your healthy lifestyle and diet with your cravings, desires and that impossible need for a bit of chocolate!

My 10 principles for having your cake and eating it

* I love sweet desserts. You love sweet desserts. Let's just accept that and enjoy them, but let's also try to make them as good for us as we can.

* Having established our desire for puddings, let's still try to stay true to giving our bodies the best nutrition possible. Food is the one thing that gives us health. There are many things that take our health away, like drinking, smoking and a sedentary lifestyle. But food is one of the things which we can control and which can actually make us stay healthy. Although desserts are usually classed as 'naughty', we all enjoy a treat once in a while, so we could say that they are good for our soul. Also, many ingredients used in my desserts still offer a good balance of nutritional benefits.

* Sugar is not always the enemy! Although we need to watch the amount of sugar we eat, it is not considered as bad for us as, say, saturated fat. Obviously sugar is high in calories, so we need to watch the quantities we eat, but a little sugar can give us a lift with immediate energy levels. There's no pretending; it's a fact that too much sugar is bad for us, but as it's also something that we crave, I believe that it is better to regulate how we use sugar and in what amounts to ensure healthy sugar levels, healthy weight and a healthy brain function. All my children are lucky to be very active and they all struggle to maintain a healthy weight, therefore, as long as they have had a good-sized nutritional meal with plenty of fresh vegetables, I am very happy for them to enjoy a homemade dessert that will satisfy their cravings and give them the extra vitamins they need from any added fruit.

* Although these are the healthiest possible desserts, they should still be looked upon as a treat! Portion size is very important. It's no

good making a healthier version of a cake if you eat the whole thing in one go! Take note of the portion size guides I have given on each recipe where possible. So even though we are going to accept that a little sugar and fat is fine in a dessert we are not going to eat a huge portion, everyday – are we? If you do get carried away and have a few too many portions, don't panic – just go for a lovely long walk and give thanks for the energy that delicious dessert has given you!

* A little note on dairy produce. You will notice that many of my dessert recipes either contain some low-fat dairy produce or are served with some. This was a conscious decision on my part, as including some low-fat dairy products into your diet is really important for your general health. Calcium is essential for healthy bones. It is also important for muscle contraction, blood vessel expansion and contraction, secretion of hormones and enzymes, transmitting impulses throughout the nervous system and normal blood clotting. So, it's pretty important!

* A study into the health benefits of milk and dairy produce commissioned by The British Heart Foundation showed that consuming milk and dairy products can massively reduce the risk of cardiovascular disease. So, while we often focus on the value of dairy foods for healthy bones and teeth in the young and elderly, this study reminds us of the importance of including dairy foods in our diet throughout our life. Dairy products can help our heart health at any age, but it's important to ensure they are low fat. So often, people following a healthy eating plan concentrate heavily on the fish, chicken fruit and vegetables, and they forget about dairy. And, in the past, heart patients especially have been warned away from dairy foods, but now it seems that common sense and balance prevail and as long as you stick to the low-fat varieties, a little dairy will do you good.

* 1 egg is an oeuf! Or is it? Contrary to common belief, your body does not absorb cholesterol from eggs. If you are on a low cholesterol diet, eggs are not a problem in this respect. Eggs do contain up to 5 grams of fat in the yolk, so this certainly has to be considered, but as far as cholesterol is concerned, eggs are not the enemy. Nutrition scientists have found that eggs are one of the most nutrient-dense foods available and are recommending that we eat at least one egg a day to get the optimum benefits. In the study, to be published in the journal 'Nutrition and Food Science', researchers discovered that eggs can play an important role in maintaining health as well as help with weight loss and dieting. The study discovered that, despite being low in calories, eggs are a rich source of protein and are packed with essential nutrients thought vital to good health, particularly vitamin D, vitamin B12 and selenium. The report also confirms that among protein foods, eggs contain the richest mix of essential amino acids, which is crucial for children, adolescents and young adults since a balance of amino acids is required for proper growth and repair. So, that proves that an egg a day keeps the doctor away!

* Fruit, fruit and more fruit. Fresh fruit is the best starting point for any dessert because of its generally sweet flavour, juicy nature, bright colour and nutritional content. So, even if you are making a dish that doesn't contain fruit, serve a side portion of fresh fruit with it to make sure you're making the most of your treat!

* Make substitutions! If you have a favourite family recipe, try to make some substitutions to make it more healthy. If you have a dessert recipe that contains butter, one of the first things you can do is use a low-fat, heart-healthy spread instead. There are wonderful heart-healthy products available that are suitable for baking, give great results

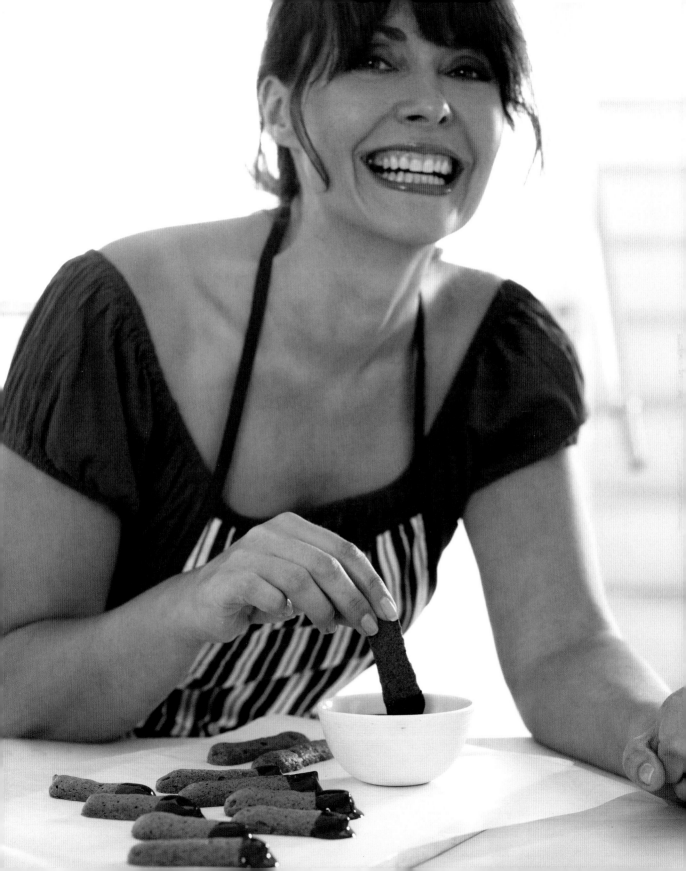

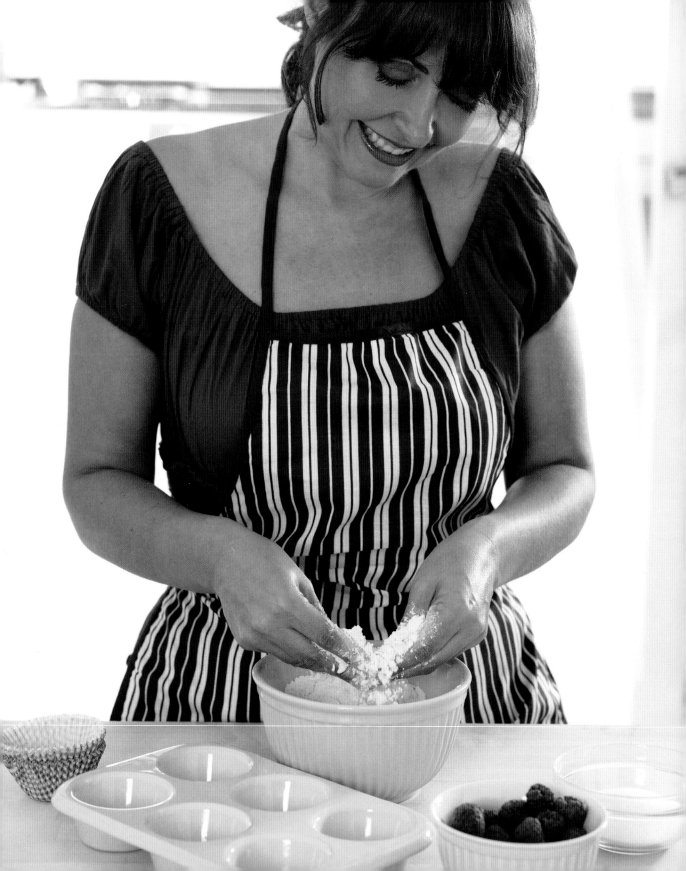

and contain only half the saturated fat of butter. It is also sometimes possible to substitute the fat in cakes for another 'wet' ingredient, such as apple sauce (see page 185) or prune purée. This will be a trial-and-error scenario for you, but do be brave and give it a go: with just a little tweaking here and there, you can produce an old favourite with half the fat. And if you come up with a really great recipe, send it to me!

* Try cutting the sugar content in a recipe in half as this often works and will just cut down on the sweetness – obviously! Or you can swap the sugar for one of the sugar substitute products on the market. I actually prefer to keep my recipes as natural as possible, so I don't use artificial sweeteners.

Why all the fruit?

Good nutrition is key to living a long and healthy life. Increasingly we are receiving poor nutrition from ready-meals, fast food and processed foods. These foods contain little, or no nutritional value, and are usually loaded with salt, hydrogenated fats and sugar. Poor nutrition can lead to various health problems in the short and long term, and make you feel tired, lethargic, and miserable too.

Nutritional Value of Fruit

Fruit is so nutritious, that we can almost live off it. A diet that is packed with plenty of fruit and nuts will be rich in protein, calcium and vitamins, which is essential for a healthy lifestyle.

Most fruit is naturally low in fat, sodium, and calories. What's more, they don't contain cholesterol, but are packed full of vitamins and minerals – the right nutrients your body needs. These nutrients include potassium, dietary fibre, vitamin C and folate (folic acid).

Potassium

Diets rich in potassium will contribute to a healthy blood pressure and a reduced risk of developing kidney stones. Fruits that contain potassium include bananas, plums, prunes, peaches, apricots and oranges.

Dietary Fibre

Regular amounts of dietary fibre help reduce blood cholesterol levels and may lower the risk of heart disease. It is also important in maintaining regular bowel movements. Fibre helps reduce constipation and therefore reduce the amount of toxins exposed to the bowel for any length of time. All fruits contain dietary fibre, but fruit juice doesn't, so you will need to eat the whole fruit to get this nutritional benefit.

Vitamin C

Vitamin C is essential for the growth and repair of body tissues. It helps heal cuts and wounds, and keeps teeth and gums healthy. It is also a powerful antioxidant that neutralises free radicals in the body. Fruits that contain vitamin C include oranges, mangoes, apples and grapes.

Folate (folic acid)

Folate helps the body form red blood cells. It is especially important for pregnant women, as folate has been proven to help prevent foetal defects from developing, such as spina bifida. Fruits that contain folate include oranges, bananas and kiwi fruit.

Antioxidants in fruit

Free radicals and antioxidants are both terms used to describe groups of vitamins, minerals and elements that help to gather up and destroy all the bad bugs and boost growth of the good bugs. Therefore when a fruit is considered high in free radicals or antioxidants, this means that it will help protect your immune system, guard against certain cancers and help boost your general good health.

Protein from Fruit

The body makes proteins to create muscles, tendons, ligaments, hair and nails. Proteins are also important in the make-up of enzymes, genes and hormones. Fruits that contain protein include: dates, avocados, figs, peanuts, almonds, Brazil nuts, and walnuts.

Fats from Fruit

Most of the fat in the Western diet is bad fat – saturated and hydrogenated fats – that increases our risk of developing heart disease and cancers. Some fat is good fat, however, and these fats contain essential fatty acids (which are the fats that are needed to help our body function rather than the type of fat that acts as a fuel which we burn for energy) and vitamins that help our bodies stay healthy. Fat improves the body's absorption of vitamins A, D and E. Fruits that contain essential fatty acids include olives, avocados, and nuts and seeds. It's also important to note that all my recipes use a low-saturated-fat, heart-healthy spread instead of butter.

So, although most people will find a diet that consists exclusively of fruit and nuts a little extreme, it shows that they contain much of what we need to live a healthy, happy life. Fruits are packed full of vitamins, minerals, essential fatty acids and proteins, and don't contain all the bad nutrition that can contribute to obesity, diabetes, Alzheimer's, and cancer. So why not take a look at your eating habits over the space of a week and add the odd healthy dessert along with extra fruit. It won't just make you feel better; it could save your life.

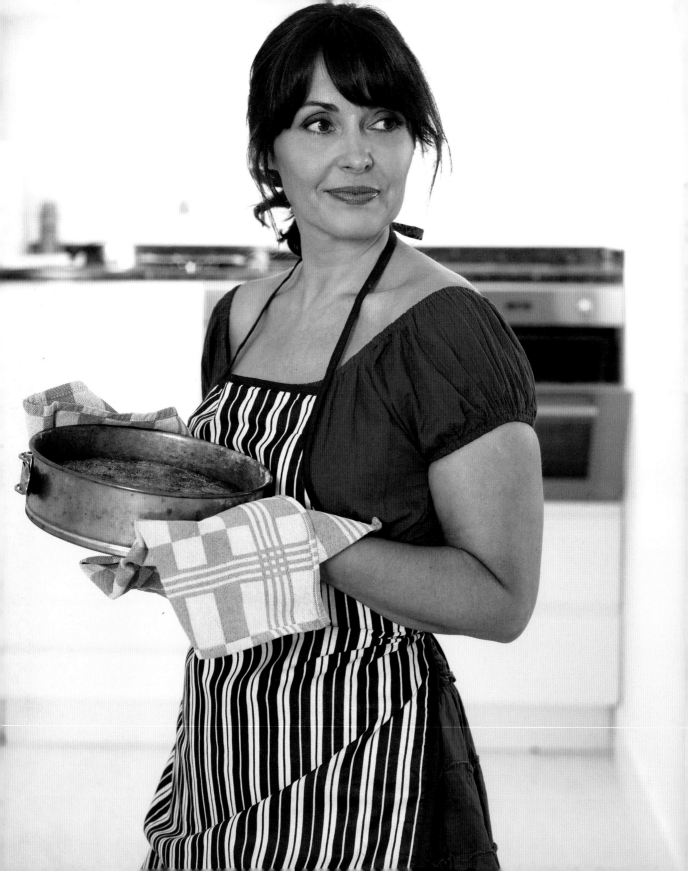

LARGE CAKES

Pistachio & Yogurt Cake

This fabulous recipe uses light olive oil and low-fat yogurt instead of butter, so keeping the fat content healthy and low. Very simple to make, this cake is beautiful served with a side order of fruit and a dollop or topping of low-fat crème fraîche or Greek yogurt.

SERVES 10

light olive oil or low-fat
  spread, for oiling
  or greasing
140g (5oz) shelled,
  unsalted pistachio nuts
4 eggs
175g (6oz) caster sugar
150g (5½oz) plain low-
  fat yogurt
75ml (3fl oz) light olive oil
115g (4oz) self-raising flour

1 Preheat the oven to 160°C/315°F/Gas mark 2–3.

2 Oil a 23cm (9in) springform cake tin with a little light olive oil or use some low-fat spread.

3 Start by finely grinding the pistachios in a food processor, then set aside.

4 Using a free-standing electric mixer, beat the eggs and the sugar together until very pale and thick. This will take about 5 minutes, so be patient with it!

5 Next, gently mix in the yogurt and olive oil.

6 Now, sift in the flour and fold in using a spatula, then add the ground pistachios.

7 Pour the mixture into the prepared tin and bake for 40 minutes or until a skewer inserted into the centre of the cake comes out clean. Allow to cool in the tin for 10 minutes, then turn out onto a wire rack to cool.

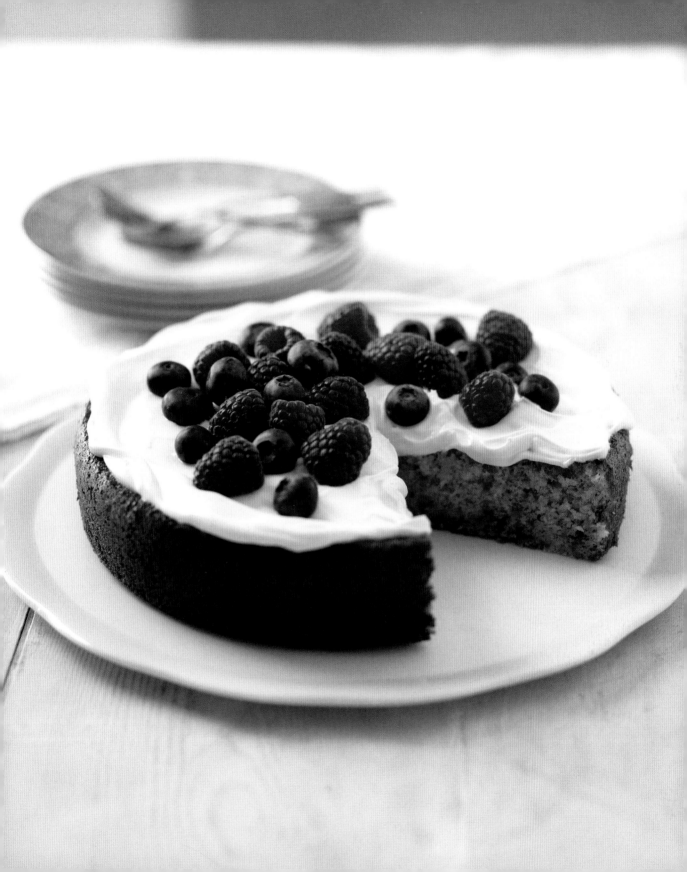

Angel Food Cake with Lemon Icing

A fat-free cake that looks seriously impressive! Serve on the day it is made with lots of sweet and colourful fruit. This recipe makes one large cake, so it is ideal for when you have a house full of guests. You will need a 25cm (10in) non-stick Bundt tin for this cake, which is available from good kitchen shops.

SERVES 12-16

12 egg whites
1¼ tsp cream of tartar
½ tsp lemon juice
grated zest of
 1 unwaxed lemon
1 tsp vanilla extract
190g (6¾oz) icing sugar
135g (4¾oz) plain flour

For the icing
juice of ½ lemon
3 tbsp clear,
 runny honey
8 tbsp icing sugar

To decorate
grated lemon zest
fresh mint sprigs

1 Preheat the oven to 180°C/350°F/Gas mark 4.

2 Using a free-standing electric mixer, whisk the egg whites and cream of tartar together until the mixture is frothy but not too stiff.

3 Next, add the lemon juice, grated lemon zest and vanilla extract, and continue to whisk while adding the icing sugar, a bit at a time. Carry on until stiff peaks form and the egg whites are nicely glossy.

4 Now, the flour needs to be sifted and added to the egg white mixture. Try to add a little height while sifting the flour over the mixture, as this will make your cake lighter. Use a spatula or large metal spoon to carefully and quickly fold in the flour until incorporated. Do not beat or overmix. Limit yourself to 16 turns of the spoon!

5 Pour the mixture into a 25cm (10in) non-stick Bundt cake tin and bake for 30–40 minutes until the top is brown and a skewer inserted halfway between the inner and outer wall of the tin comes out clean.

recipe continues...

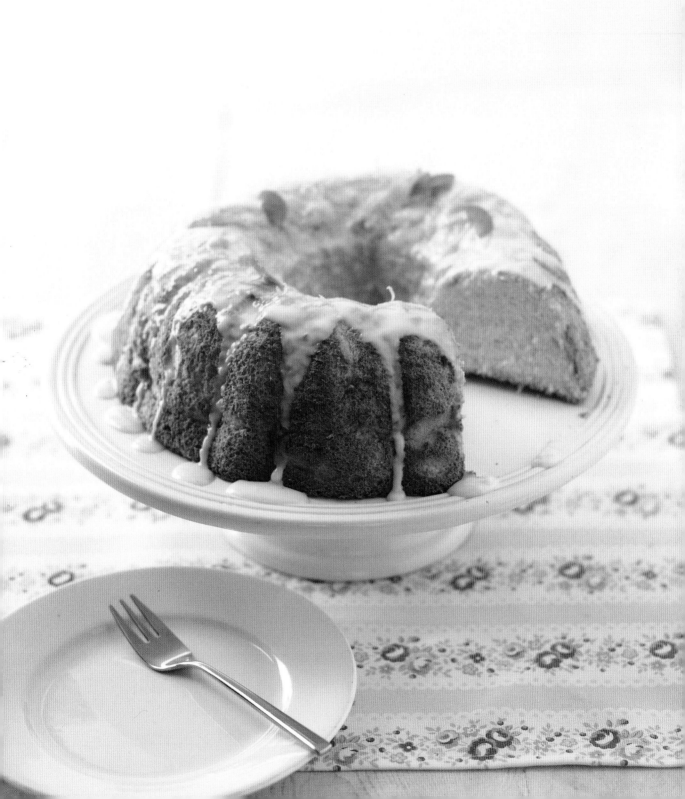

6   Don't turn the cake out, simply turn the tin upside down on top of a wire rack and leave the cake to cool inside the tin for about an hour.

7   Now, carefully use a plastic spatula to loosen the cake around the sides and middle, then release the cake and place on a serving plate.

8   For the icing, simply mix the lemon juice, honey and icing sugar together and pour over the cake just before serving. Decorate with lemon zest and mint sprigs.

Low-fat Ginger Cake

If it's holiday time, make this to fill your house with festive smells. If it's not holiday time, make it anyway! This cake is easy to make, delicious and low in fat – enjoy a delicious piece of this ginger cake guilt-free any time.

SERVES 9

light cooking spray,
  for coating
200g (7oz) dark
  muscovado sugar
1 egg
60ml (2fl oz) light olive oil
125ml (4fl oz) low-fat
  buttermilk
200g (7oz) plain flour
1 tsp ground ginger
1 tsp ground cinnamon
½ tsp baking powder

TIP
Feel free to dust the top of the cake with a little mixture of icing sugar and cocoa powder.

1   Preheat the oven to 180°C/350°F/Gas mark 4.

2   Spray a 20cm (8in) square cake tin with light cooking spray and line the base with baking parchment.

3   In a large bowl, mix the sugar, egg and olive oil together until smooth. Now, add the buttermilk and combine well.

4   Next, sift the flour, ground ginger, cinnamon and baking powder into the wet ingredients and mix with a wooden spoon. Don't overmix.

5   Pour the mixture into the prepared tin and bake for 25–30 minutes or until a skewer inserted into the centre of the cake comes out clean. Allow to cool in the tin for 5 minutes, then turn out onto a wire rack to cool. Once cold, cut into squares to serve.

Fruity Fruit Cake

Now don't expect a very sweet and heavy traditional fruit cake with this recipe. Made with low-fat spread and only a tiny amount of sugar, this cake is wonderfully light and naturally sweetened by the dried fruit.

SERVES 10

low-fat spread,
  for greasing
150g (5½oz) mixed
  dried fruit
20g (¾oz) pecan nuts,
  hazelnuts or
  walnuts, chopped
100g (3½oz) self-raising
  flour
100g (3½oz) low-fat,
  heart-healthy spread
50g (1¾oz) dark
  muscovado sugar
2 eggs

1 Preheat the oven to 180°C/350°F/Gas mark 4.

2 Grease a 20cm (8in) loose-bottomed cake tin with low-fat spread.

3 In a bowl, combine the dried fruit and chopped nuts along with 1 tablespoon of the flour. Set aside.

4 In another bowl, beat the low-fat spread and the sugar together. You might need to squash the clumps of sugar with the back of a fork.

5 Now, add the eggs and beat into the sugar mixture. Using a wooden spoon is fine.

6 Next, add the remaining flour and mix well.

7 Finally, add the flour-coated fruit and nuts and stir to combine.

8 Pour the mixture into the prepared tin and bake for 18–20 minutes or until a skewer inserted into the centre comes out clean. Allow to cool in the tin for 5 minutes, then turn out onto a wire rack to cool.

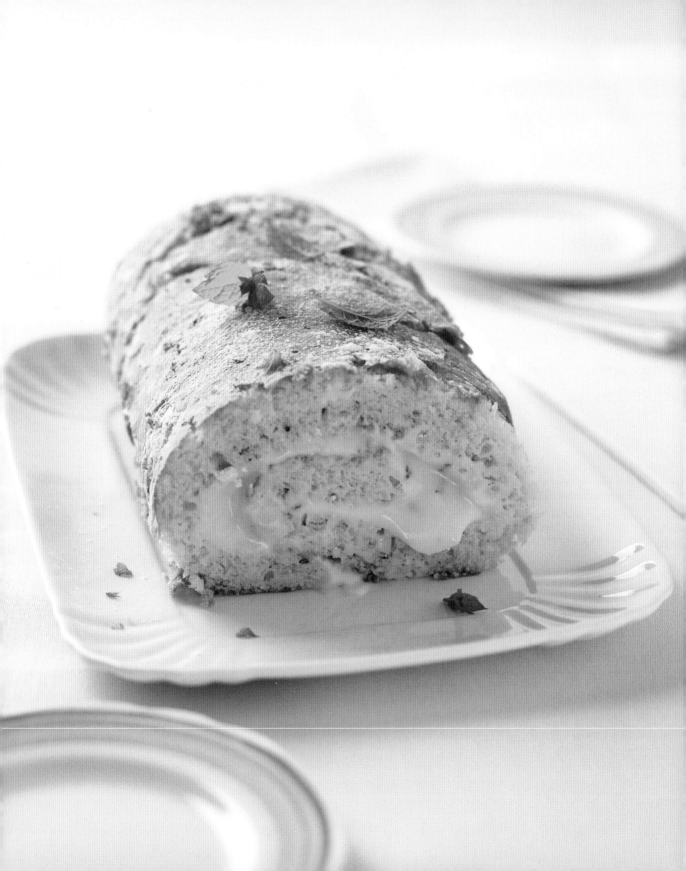

Mint, Caraway & Lemon Roulade

This is an impressive-looking, delicious and light roulade that contains only half the fat compared to one made with butter and full-fat cream cheese filling. This roulade is best eaten on the day it is made.

SERVES 8

6 eggs
175g (6oz) golden
  caster sugar
175g (6oz) self-raising
  flour
grated zest of
  1 unwaxed lemon
1 tsp caraway seeds,
  lightly crushed
55g (2oz) low-fat heart-
  healthy spread, melted
icing sugar, for sprinkling
1 fresh mint sprig,
  to decorate

For the filling
200g (7oz) low-fat,
  cream cheese
juice of ½ lemon
275g (10oz) lemon curd
6 fresh lemon-mint or
  mint leaves

1 Preheat the oven to 200°C/400°F/Gas mark 6.

2 Line a 27 x 40cm (11¼ x 16in) Swiss roll tin with non-stick baking parchment.

3 Using a free-standing electric mixer, whisk the eggs and caster sugar together until the mixture is very light and fluffy and almost doubled in volume. This will take about 5 minutes, so be patient with it!

4 Now, using either a spatula or a large metal spoon, fold in the flour, grated lemon zest, crushed caraway seeds, and melted low-fat spread. Do not overmix.

5 Pour the mixture into the prepared tin and bake, checking it after 12 minutes. You don't want too much colour on the sponge, so keep a close eye on it for a maximum of 16 minutes until it is light and springy to the touch. As soon as you can see that the sponge is cooked in the middle but not browning around the edges, remove from the oven and turn the sponge out onto a sheet of non-stick greaseproof paper sprinkled with a little icing sugar.

6 Allow to cool in the tin for 5 minutes, then turn out onto a sheet of non-stick baking parchment sprinkled with some icing sugar, and using the baking parchment, carefully roll up into a Swiss roll. Allow to cool.

recipe continues...

7   To make the filling, mix the cheese, lemon juice and
lemon curd together in a bowl.

8   Now, very finely slice the lemon-mint or mint leaves
and mix these into the lemon curd mixture.

9   Only when the sponge has completely cooled,
carefully unroll and spread the inside of the sponge
with the lemon and mint cream. Now, re-roll the
cake using the baking parchment to help keep it
all together. Place on a serving dish, dust with a
little icing sugar and top with the mint sprig.

Courgette Loaf

These sweet loaves make a perfect mid-morning or mid-afternoon snack. The
bulk of the courgettes keep the calories lower, and with no butter added, a
modest slice of this is a lovely healthy treat.

MAKES 2 LOAVES
EACH SERVING 10

low-fat spread,
  for greasing
3 medium eggs
240ml (8½fl oz) light
  olive oil
480g (17oz) caster sugar
720g (1lb 9oz) plain flour,
  sifted
2 tsp baking powder, sifted
1 tsp ground cinnamon
480g (17oz) courgettes,
  coarsely grated
2 tsp vanilla extract
50g (1¾ oz) chopped
  walnuts

1   Preheat the oven to 180°C/350°F/Gas mark 4.

2   Grease 2 x 900g (2lb) loaf tins with low-fat spread
and line the bases with baking parchment.

3   Using a hand whisk, mix the eggs and olive oil
together in a large bowl.

4   Next, add the caster sugar and whisk for a further
3 minutes.

5   Now, fold in the sifted flour, baking powder and
cinnamon with a large metal spoon, then add the
grated courgettes, vanilla extract and chopped
walnuts and mix well.

6   Pour the cake mixture evenly between the prepared
loaf tins and bake for 1 hour or until risen and golden.
Serve warm or cold with a lovely cup of tea!

Butter-free Fudge Cake

In this recipe I have used homemade apple sauce instead of butter, making it a half-fat version compared to a usual fudge cake. This cake is lovely served just as it is, but if you want to cover the top with a chocolate frosting, take a look at the frosting recipes on pages 182–183.

SERVES 9

light cooking spray, for coating
85g (3oz) wholemeal plain flour
25g (1oz) oatbran
30g (1oz) cocoa powder
100g (3½oz) dark brown sugar
100g (3½oz) caster sugar
1 tsp bicarbonate of soda
175g (6oz) homemade apple sauce (see page 185)
3 tbsp vegetable oil or light olive oil
2 tbsp strong black coffee
1 egg white, beaten
1 tsp vanilla extract

TIP
This cake is delicious served with a squirt of Raspberry Coulis (see page 184).

1 Preheat the oven to 170°C/325°F/Gas mark 3.

2 Spray a 20cm (8in) square cake tin with light cooking spray and line the base with non-stick baking parchment.

3 Place the flour, oatbran, cocoa, both sugars and the bicarbonate of soda in a medium-sized bowl and stir to mix well.

4 Now, combine the apple sauce, oil, coffee, beaten egg white and vanilla extract and stir to mix. Add the apple sauce mixture to the flour mixture and combine well.

5 Pour the cake mixture into the prepared tin and bake for about 25 minutes or until the top springs back when lightly touched and a wooden skewer inserted into the centre of the cake comes out clean. Allow to cool in the tin for 5 minutes, then turn out onto a wire rack to cool.

Almond & Hazelnut Gateau

I love making this nutty, butter-free gateau. It's incredibly light and works fabulously with a thick layer of fat-free frosting on top. Hazelnuts and almonds are a great source of vitamin E, dietary fibre, heart-healthy B vitamins and 'good fats', and the eggs add the protein. This cake is best eaten on the day it is made.

SERVES 8
(LARGER SLICES ALLOWED, AS IS THIS IS A LOVELY LOW-FAT CAKE)

light cooking spray,
  for coating
4 medium eggs
100g (3½oz) caster sugar
5½ tbsp plain flour
50g (1¾oz) ground almonds
50g (1¾oz) ground
  hazelnuts
50g (1¾oz) flaked almonds

To decorate
frosting of your choice
  (see pages 182–183)
raspberries
plain dark chocolate
  scrapings

1 Preheat the oven to 190°C/375°F/Gas mark 5.

2 Spray two 20cm (8in) sandwich tins with light cooking spray to make the cake easy to turn out.

3 Using a free-standing electric mixer, whisk the eggs and sugar together until the mixture is pale, fluffy and doubled in volume. Be patient, as this will take about 5 minutes.

4 Now, sift in the flour from a good height. Add the ground almonds and hazelnuts and fold in with a large, clean metal spoon using as few strokes as possible.

5 Tip the mixture gently into the prepared tins and sprinkle with the flaked almonds.

6 Bake for 12 minutes until well risen and springy to the touch. Allow to cool in the tins for 5 minutes, then turn out and cool on a wire rack.

7 Cover one cake with delicious low-fat frosting and maybe some raspberries. Place the second cake on top. Decorate with more low-fat frosting, raspberries and dark chocolate scrapings.

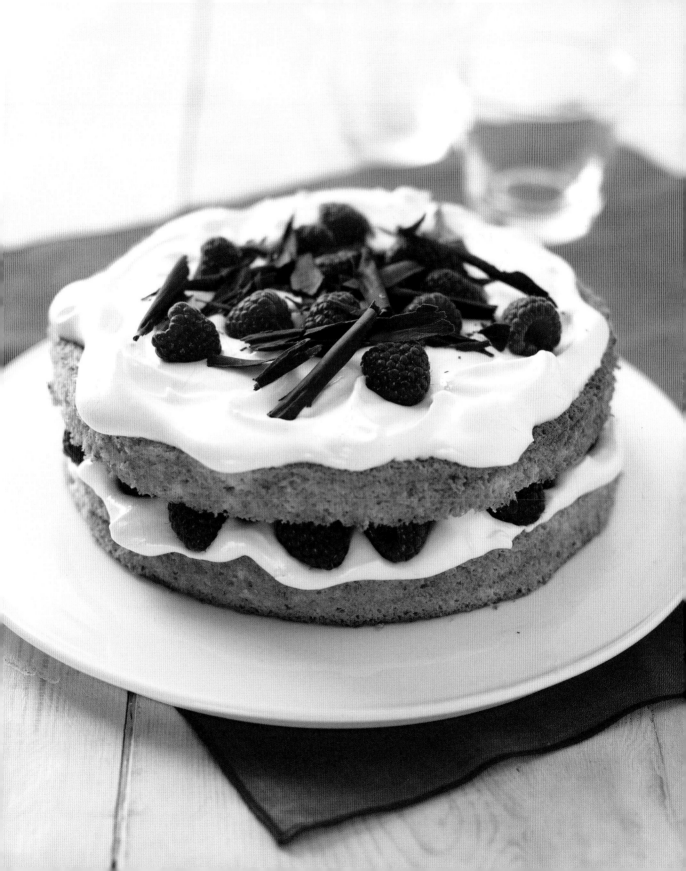

Chocolate Cake with Spicy Pears

This butter- and flour-free cake has a lovely light texture and great flavour. Make sure you use best quality plain dark chocolate, as this will contain less fat and sugar and gives a better flavour. Cook the pears a day ahead and chill in the refrigerator overnight. The cake is best eaten on the day it is baked.

SERVES 4

For the cake
low-fat spread,
    for greasing
110g (4oz) caster sugar,
    plus 1 tbsp for dusting
1 tbsp plain flour,
    for dusting
110g (4oz) bitter dark
    chocolate, chopped
4 eggs, separated
70g (2½oz) cornflour
icing sugar, sifted,
    for dusting
low-fat crème fraîche,
    to serve

ingredients continue...

1 Start by making the pears. Put 150ml (5fl oz) water, the sugar and honey into a large heavy saucepan and mix together over a low heat until the sugar has dissolved completely. Bring to the boil, then add the cloves, peppercorns, cinnamon, ginger and orange zest and cook for 10 minutes, uncovered, or until slightly thickened and syrupy.

2 Allow the syrup to cool slightly, then mix in the wine and lemon juice.

3 Peel the pears, leaving the stems intact and stud each pear with 2 cloves. Immediately submerge the pears into the syrup to prevent discolouring. Bring slowly to the boil, then reduce the heat and simmer gently for 15 minutes. Remove the pan from the heat and allow the pears to cool completely in the syrup. Refrigerate overnight.

4 The next day, make the cake. Preheat the oven to 180°C/350°F/Gas mark 4.

5 Grease a 23cm (9in) cake tin with low-fat spread and line the base with a disc of greaseproof paper. Dust lightly with the 1 tablespoon sugar and then the 1 tablespoon flour, tapping out the excess.

recipe continues...

For the spicy pears
85g (3oz) caster sugar
2 tbsp clear, runny honey
4 cloves
10 black peppercorns
1 cinnamon stick
1 x 2.5cm (1in) piece of
    fresh ginger, peeled
    and sliced
thinly pared zest of
    1 orange
290 ml (10fl oz) Muscat
    wine
juice of ½ lemon
4 firm, ripe pears
8 cloves

6 Put the chocolate into a heatproof bowl set over a saucepan of simmering water, making sure the base of the bowl isn't touching the water, and stir continuously until the chocolate has melted, then remove from the heat.

7 In a separate bowl, beat the egg yolks with all but 1 tablespoon of the caster sugar until pale and creamy. Mix the cornflour into the egg yolk mixture, then pour in the melted chocolate and mix thoroughly.

8 Using a free-standing electric mixer, whisk the egg whites with the remaining 1 tablespoon sugar until shiny and stiff. Using a large metal spoon, fold the egg whites into the egg and chocolate mixture and pour into the prepared tin.

9 Bake the cake in the centre of the oven for 20–25 minutes. Allow to cool in the tin for 10 minutes, then turn out onto a wire rack to cool.

10 Lightly dust the cake with icing sugar just before serving with the well-chilled pears and a scoop of low-fat crème fraîche.

Beetroot & Chocolate Cake

Chocolate and beetroot are an unusual combination but one that works well. Using light olive oil instead of butter and taking into account the antioxidants and potassium contained in the beetroot and dark chocolate, this cake is perfect for the most health-conscious, sweet teeth around.

SERVES 12

low-fat spread, for greasing
50g (1¾oz) cocoa powder
175g (6oz) plain flour
1½ tsp baking powder
200g (7oz) caster sugar
250g (9oz) cooked
   beetroot in juice
3 eggs
200ml (7fl oz) light olive oil
100g (3½oz) good-quality
   plain dark chocolate,
   finely chopped
170g (6oz) icing sugar
low-fat crème fraîche,
   to serve

TIP
Remember that it is important to include some low-fat dairy into your diet to support your bones and circulatory system, so a dollop of low-fat crème fraîche is a perfect accompaniment to a small slice of cake.

1 Preheat the oven to 180°C/350°F/Gas mark 4.

2 Grease a 23cm (9in) loose-bottomed cake tin with a little low-fat spread and line the base with baking parchment.

3 Sift the cocoa, flour and baking powder into a large mixing bowl. Add the sugar and mix with a wooden spoon to combine.

4 Drain the beetroot, reserving the juice, then put the beetroot in a food processor along with the eggs and the olive oil and blitz until smooth.

5 Now, make a well in the centre of the dry ingredients and, using a wooden spoon, beat in the beetroot mixture, a bit at a time to form a smooth batter.

6 Next, add the chopped chocolate and combine well. Pour the mixture into the prepared cake tin and bake for 40–45 minutes or until a skewer inserted into the centre of the cake comes out clean. Allow to cool in the tin for 5 minutes, then turn out onto a wire rack and cool.

7 To make the icing, simply mix the icing sugar with a little of the reserved beetroot juice to make a deep purple pourable icing. Drizzle the icing over the cake and serve with a dollop of low-fat crème fraîche.

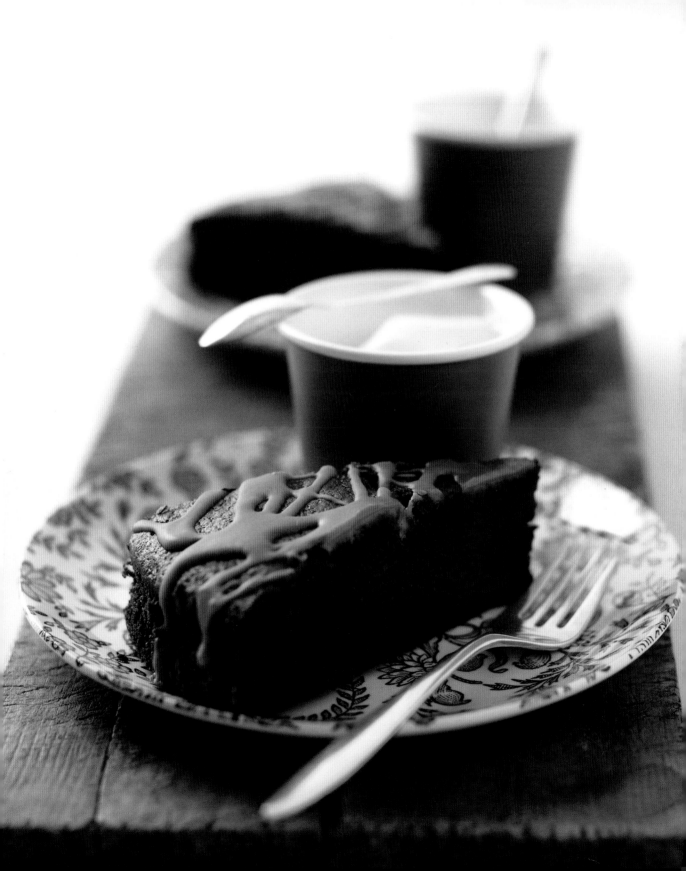

Fat-free Chocolate Fudge Brownies

You can enjoy these brownies guilt-free. I have substituted the butter with apple sauce. You can make your own apple sauce, of course, or you can buy it in some health food shops. A friend of mine uses baby apple sauce, which makes sense because this is completely natural with no added sugar.

SERVES 9

low-fat spread,
  for greasing
3 egg whites
175g (6oz) self-raising flour
85g (3oz) cocoa powder,
  plus extra for dusting
225g (8oz) caster sugar
55g (2oz) chopped walnuts
  or pecan nuts
1 tsp vanilla extract
70g (2½oz) unsweetened
  apple sauce
  (see page 185)

1 Preheat the oven to 160°C/315°F/Gas mark 2-3.

2 Grease a 20cm (8in) square cake tin with low-fat spread.

3 Using a free-standing electric mixer, whisk the egg whites until doubled in volume and stiff peaks form.

4 In a separate bowl, sift the flour and cocoa powder together, then mix in the sugar and the chopped nuts. (I quite like a mixture of walnuts and pecans).

5 Finally, add the vanilla extract, apple sauce and the stiff egg whites and fold in gently using a large metal spoon or spatula. Do not overmix.

6 Pour the mixture into the prepared tin and bake for 20-25 minutes or until the edges are firmly set and the centre is almost set. Allow to cool in the tin for 5 minutes then turn out onto a wire rack to cool.

7 Once cold, dust with cocoa powder, then cut into squares and serve.

Nutty Banana Cake

This is a delicious and healthy, fruity nutty cake and just so easy to make! I use apple sauce instead of fat and wholemeal flour to boost the fibre content. Try to use very ripe bananas. Did you know that you can freeze ripe bananas to keep them safe until you have enough to make your dish? Freeze them (see p153), then thaw out for a couple of hours, peel and use as normal.

SERVES 12

low-fat spread,
  for greasing
6 tbsp unsweetened
  apple sauce
  (see page 185)
100g (3½oz) clear,
  runny honey
2 eggs
3 ripe bananas,
  mashed up well
  with a fork
1 tsp vanilla extract
200g (7oz) wholemeal
  self-raising flour
1 tsp bicarbonate of soda
50g (1¾oz) chopped
  walnuts

1 Preheat the oven to 160°C/315°F/Gas mark 2–3.

2 Grease a 23 x 12cm (9 x 5in) loaf tin with low-fat spread and line the base with non-stick baking parchment.

3 In a large bowl, mix the apple sauce and honey together.

4 Next, add the eggs and beat well, then stir in the mashed bananas and vanilla extract, making sure everything is well combined.

5 Stir in the flour. Put the bicarbonate of soda into a cup and add 4 tablespoons of hand-hot water. Stir to mix and pour immediately into the batter, stirring quickly and well.

6 Finally, stir in the chopped walnuts and pour the mixture into the prepared tin. Bake for 55–60 minutes. Allow to cool in the tin for 5 minutes, then turn out onto a wire rack to cool for 30 minutes before slicing.

TIP
If your bananas are not quite ripe enough, peel and pop in the microwave for 20 seconds and they'll be perfect!

Low-fat Frosted Carrot Cake

This is a very easy recipe that my whole family enjoys. I have added a little ground ginger just because I love the combination, but feel free to omit it if you prefer. I love this cake without the frosting just as much as with it, but if you are using the frosting, add it just before serving, as it will soak into the cake if left for too long.

SERVES 8

low-fat spread,
 for greasing
2 medium eggs
175g (6oz) dark
 muscovado sugar
75ml (3fl oz) light olive oil
200g (7oz) wholemeal
 self-raising flour
1 level tsp bicarbonate
 of soda
1 level tsp baking powder
1 tsp ground ginger
 (optional)
2 tsp mixed spice
grated zest 1 lemon
200g (7oz) carrots, peeled
 and coarsely grated
175g (6oz) sultanas
60ml (2fl oz) pineapple
 juice
grated zest 1 orange

For the frosting
225g (8oz) Quark (virtually
 fat-free soft cheese)
55g (2oz) icing sugar
2 tbsp lemon juice

1   Preheat the oven to 180°C/350°F/Gas mark 4.

2   Grease a 20cm (8in) cake tin with low-fat spread and line the base with non-stick baking parchment.

3   Using an electric whisk, combine the eggs, sugar and olive oil together.

4   Next, sift the flour, bicarbonate of soda , baking powder, ground ginger (if using) and the mixed spice into the egg mixture. If there are any bits left in the sieve from the flour, just pour these in. Mix together using a large metal spoon, then add the lemon zest, grated carrots, sultanas and pineapple juice and stir to combine but don't overmix.

5   Finally, pour the mixture into the prepared tin and bake for 35–40 minutes until well risen and a skewer inserted into the centre of the cake comes out clean. Allow to cool in the tin for at least 5 minutes, then turn out onto a wire rack to cool.

6   To make the frosting, simply mix the Quark, icing sugar and lemon juice together in a bowl. When the cake is completely cold, use a spatula to spread the frosting over the cake and decorate with grated orange zest, then cut into squares and serve.

TIP
It is a good idea to make the frosting ahead of time and leave to chill in the refrigerator for at least an hour before using.

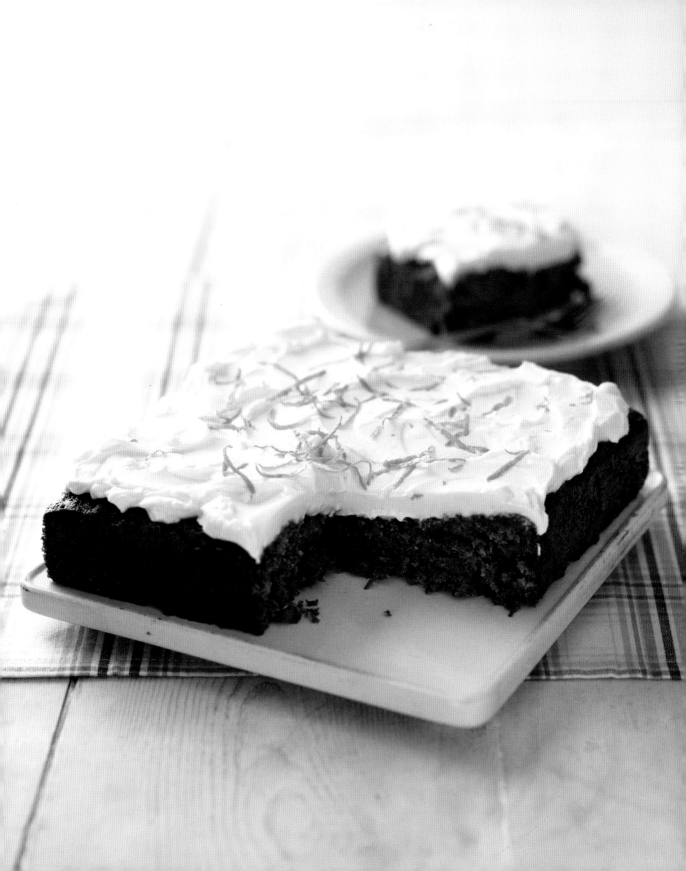

German Honey Cake

This is a delicious, old-fashioned cake. I love it because it uses olive oil instead of butter. Contrary to what many people believe, olive oil doesn't lose its goodness when it's heated. The only time the nutrients in olive oil would be lost are if it is heated repeatedly. This cake has a traditional, slightly spicy flavour. Once you try it, you'll know what I mean! Don't use an electric mixer for the main part of this recipe – mixing by hand is much better, but I do recommend that you use an electric whisk for the egg whites.

SERVES 12

low-fat spread, for greasing
2 tsp instant coffee granules
2 eggs, separated
85g (3oz) dark muscovado
 sugar
3 tbsp light olive oil
110g (4oz) runny honey
200g (7oz) wholemeal
 plain flour
2 teaspoons baking powder
½ tsp bicarbonate of soda
½ tsp ground cloves
½ tsp ground allspice

1 Preheat the oven to 160°C/315°F/Gas mark 2–3.

2 Grease a 20cm (8in) round loose-bottomed cake tin with low-fat spread.

3 Start by dissolving the coffee in 125ml (4fl oz) hot water, and setting aside.

4 Now, in a large bowl, beat the egg yolks and muscovado sugar together thoroughly until the mixture goes a little paler. Add the olive oil and the honey and beat until the mixture is creamy and glossy.

5 Next, sift together the flour, baking powder, bicarbonate of soda and spices. Add these dry ingredients along with the coffee to the egg and honey mixture and mix with a wooden spoon. Don't worry if it is a little lumpy – this will add to the texture. Don't beat or overmix.

6 Finally, using a free-standing electric mixer, whisk the egg whites until stiff peaks form, then using a large metal spoon or spatula, fold gently into the batter mixture. Again, be careful not to overmix. Only allow yourself 15 turns of the spoon!

7 Pour the batter into the prepared tin and bake for 35–40 minutes or until a skewer inserted into the centre of cake comes out clean. Allow to cool in the tin for 5 minutes, then turn out onto a wire rack to cool.

Low-fat Date & Walnut Block

Using the low-fat, heart-healthy spread instead of butter makes this dish healthier than a traditional version from the get-go. Wholemeal flour and dates add great fibre and the walnuts contain a host of vitamins and minerals, as well as omega-3 fatty acids, which are very important for heart and skin health. A slice of this for breakfast with a glass of fresh fruit juice will keep you going until lunch beautifully.

SERVES 9

40g (1½oz) low-fat, heart-healthy spread,
 plus extra for greasing
200g (7oz) pitted dried
 dates
I tsp bicarbonate of soda
50g (1¾oz) muscovado
 sugar
1 egg
½ tsp vanilla extract
180g (6¼oz) wholemeal
 self-raising flour
1 tsp baking powder
½ tsp mixed spice
50g (1¾oz) walnut pieces

1 Preheat the oven to 180°C/350°F/Gas mark 4.

2 Grease a 22cm (8½in) square cake tin with low-fat spread and line the base with non-stick baking parchment.

3 Place the dates in a large bowl, cover with 300ml (10fl oz) boiling water and sprinkle over the bicarbonate of soda. Leave to soak for 10 minutes, then drain the dates and reserve the soaking liquid.

4 Put the sugar, low-fat spread, egg and vanilla extract into a food processor and mix together well.

5 Now, sift the flour, baking powder and mixed spice into the food processor and add the reserved soaking liquid from the dates and blitz until well combined.

6 Finally, add the walnut pieces and the drained dates and pulse very briefly until the dates and nuts are just roughly chopped, but not blended.

7 Pour the mixture into the prepared tin and bake for 40–50 minutes until golden and a skewer inserted into the centre comes out clean. Allow to cool in the tin for 5 minutes, then turn out onto a wire rack to cool before cutting into squares to serve.

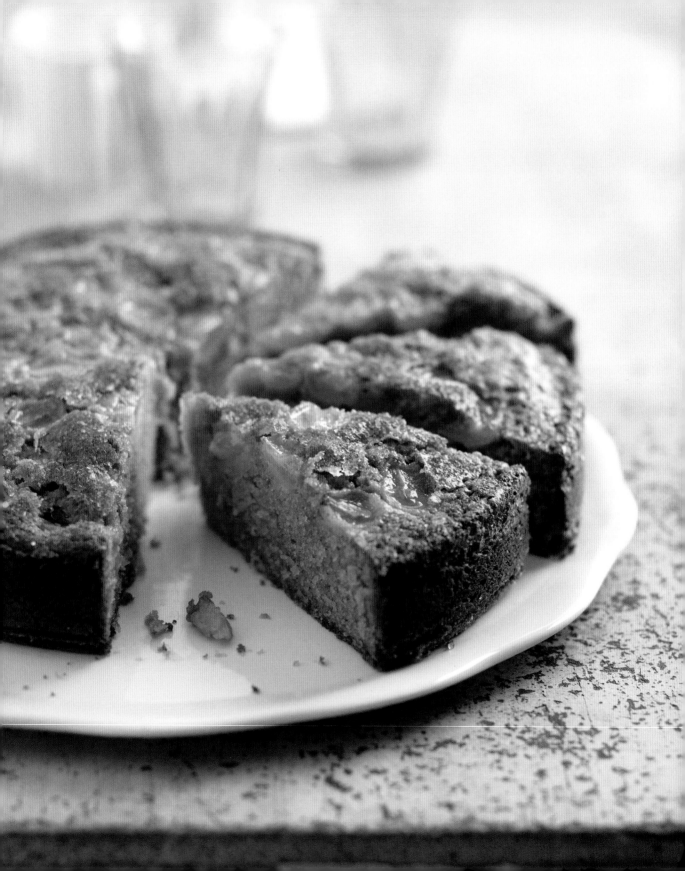

Tuscan Grape Cake

This is one of my all-time favourite cakes. Butter is replaced by a little low-fat spread and olive oil, and feel free to use extra virgin instead of light, as the cake is strong enough to take the extra flavour.

SERVES 12

225ml (8fl oz) sweet
  white wine
175ml (6fl oz) extra
  virgin olive oil,
  plus extra for oiling
225g (8oz) plain flour,
  plus 1 tbsp for dusting
200g (8oz) light
  muscovado sugar
100g (3½oz) low-fat spread
3 eggs
grated zest of 1 orange
grated zest of 1 lemon
1 tsp baking powder
175g (6oz) grapes, halved
  and deseeded
4–5 tbsp demerara sugar

TIP
This cake will store in an
airtight container for up
to 3 days.

1   Preheat the oven to 180°C/350°F/Gas mark 4.

2   Pour the wine into a small pan and bring to the boil, then lower the heat and keep simmering until the wine has reduced down to 85ml (3fl oz), about 5–10 minutes. Allow to cool.

3   Oil a 23cm (9in) loose-bottomed cake tin with olive oil, tip in 1 tablespoon of flour, then shake all over the pan until covered. Tip out any excess flour.

4   Using a wooden spoon, beat the light muscovado sugar and low-fat spread together in a bowl until creamy and well combined. Add the eggs, one at a time, then stir through the citrus zests.

5   Stir the cooled wine and olive oil together, then pour a little into the cake mixture. Stir, then fold in one-third of the flour and the baking powder. Keep alternating between adding the liquid and flour until everything has been incorporated and the mixture is smooth.

6   Spoon the cake mixture into the prepared tin, smoothing the surface with the back of the spoon. Scatter the halved grapes over the top and sprinkle over the demerara sugar. Bake for 35–40 minutes until a skewer inserted into the centre of the cake comes out clean. Allow to cool in the tin for 5 minutes, then turn out onto a wire rack to cool. Eat warm or cool.

Fat-free Strawberry Victoria Sponge

This sponge cake sounds too good to be true – but as simple as it is, it works. Use this recipe as a basis for lots of different cakes. You can jazz it up by adding different toppings, fruits and low-fat creams! The only thing I would say is that this sponge needs to be eaten on the day it is made, otherwise it goes a bit chewy! You can spread with jam and top with fresh fruit and just a sifting of icing sugar to make a delicious, guilt-free dessert. The eggs keep the cake fluffy and light, so be sure to whisk them thoroughly.

SERVES 12

light cooking spray,
  for coating
4 eggs
115g (4oz) caster sugar
115g (4oz) plain flour or
  85g (3oz) flour and
  25g (1oz) good-quality
  cocoa if you want a
  chocolate cake!

**For the fat-free
  frosting**
300g (10½oz) caster sugar
2 egg whites
1 tbsp lemon juice
3 tbsp orange juice

To decorate
I punnet of strawberries
  (about 400g/14oz)
icing sugar, for dusting

1 Preheat the oven to 180°C/350°F/Gas mark 4.

2 Spray a 20cm (8in) round cake tin with light cooking spray to make the cake easy to turn out.

3 Using a free-standing electric mixer, whisk the eggs and sugar together until the mixture is pale, fluffy and doubled in volume. Be patient, this will take about 5 minutes.

4 Now, sift in the flour and cocoa powder (if using) from a good height, and fold in with a large, clean, metal spoon using as few strokes as possible.

5 Pour the mixture gently into the prepared tin and bake for 30–35 minutes. Allow to cool in the tin for 5 minutes, then turn out onto a wire rack to cool.

   recipe continues...

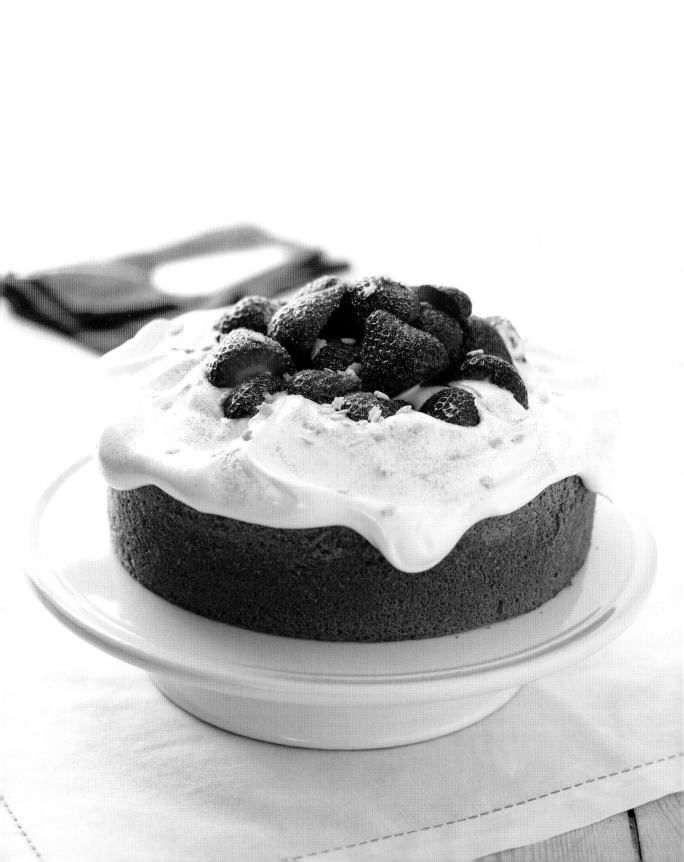

TIP
Of course, you can replace
the strawberries with any
other fruit you fancy!

6 To make the frosting, put all the ingredients into a
   large heatproof bowl set over a pan of simmering
   water and stir over the heat until all the sugar has
   completely dissolved.

7 Now, keeping the bowl over the simmering water, use
   a hand-held electric mixer to whisk the mixture until
   thickened and soft peaks form. Remove the bowl from
   the heat and continue to whisk until the mixture is cool.

8 Use a palette knife to spread the frosting over the
   cake and decorate with a pile of fresh strawberries.
   Finally, dust with icing sugar or sprinkle with any
   other pretty, edible decorations and serve.

SMALL CAKES

White Angel Wing Cupcakes

These very pretty and delicate cupcakes get eaten by my little angels in minutes! Although still containing sugar and some low-fat spread, I am always happy to let my little ones have a couple of these treats after school, knowing that they are chemical- and additive-free!

MAKES 12 CUPCAKES

175g (6oz) self-raising
  flour, sifted
1 tsp baking powder
115g (4oz) low-fat, heart-
  healthy spread
200g (7oz) caster sugar,
  divided equally into
  2 portions
2 eggs
1 tsp vanilla extract
120ml (4fl oz) skimmed milk
a pinch of cream of tartar

For the angelic
  frosting (low-fat
  cream cheese
  frosting)
450g (1lb) low-fat
  cream cheese
125g (4½oz) low-fat, heart-
  healthy spread
250g (9oz) icing sugar,
  sifted
1 tsp vanilla extract

1 Preheat the oven to 180°C/350°F/Gas mark 4.

2 Line a 12-hole muffin tin with 12 pretty paper muffin cases.

3 In a large mixing bowl, sift together the flour and baking powder and set aside.

4 Using a free-standing electric mixer, beat the low-fat spread and half of the sugar until light and fluffy.

5 Separate the eggs and set the whites aside. Add the egg yolks and vanilla extract to the sugar mixture and beat together until incorporated. Now, add the flour mixture along with the milk, a bit at a time until the mixture is smooth.

6 In another clean bowl and using a clean electric whisk, beat the egg whites until soft peaks form. At this point add the cream of tartar and the other half of the sugar and continue to whisk until stiff peaks form and the egg whites are glossy. Use a spatula to gently fold the egg whites into the cupcake mixture, but don't overmix!

7 Evenly fill the 12 muffin cases with the mixture and bake for about 18–20 minutes or until nicely browned and a cocktail stick inserted into a cupcake comes out clean. Allow to cool on a wire rack.

recipe continues...

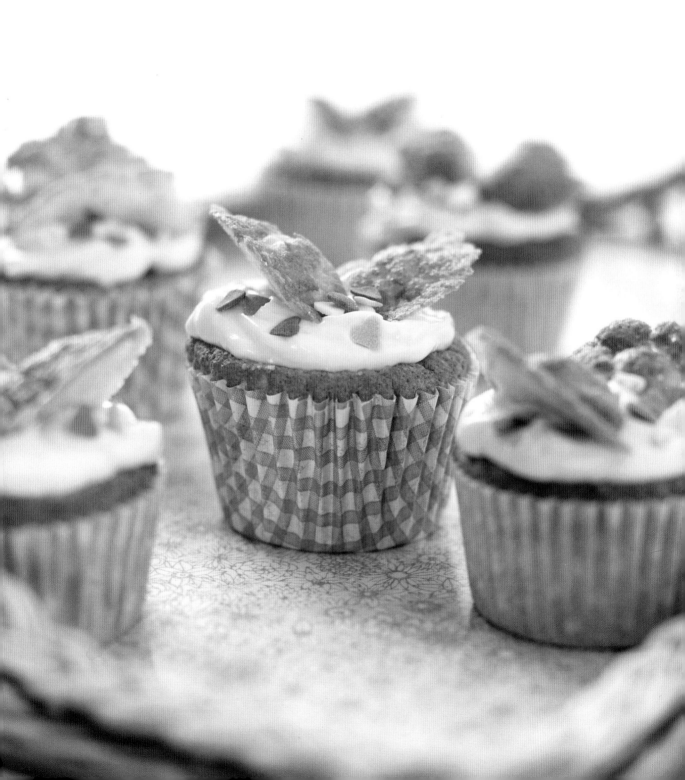

8   To make the frosting, simply mix all the ingredients together in a bowl until well combined, then cool in the refrigerator for 10 minutes before using.

9   Once the cupcakes are cool, cut out a 'lid' from the top of each cake and cut in half. Fill the hole with the frosting and place the two lid halves back on top at an angle to form the angel wings. Sprinkle with pretty, edible decorations if you like.

Prune & Oat Muffins

Prunes are a wonderful source of potassium, fibre and vitamin B6, so therefore these muffins are not only filling and energy-giving, they will give your heart health a tick in the box. They are lovely eaten either warm or cold.

MAKES 12

140g (5oz) plain flour
1 tbsp baking powder
115g (4oz) demerara sugar
140g (5oz) porridge oats
150g (5½oz) pitted prunes, chopped
6 tbsp light olive oil
2 eggs
250ml (9fl oz) low-fat buttermilk
1 tsp vanilla extract
1 tbsp porridge oats and sunflower seeds, for sprinkling

1   Preheat the oven to 200°C/350°F/Gas mark 6.

2   Line a 12-hole muffin tin with paper muffin cases.

3   Sift the flour and baking powder together into a large bowl and add the sugar, oats and chopped prunes.

4   In another bowl, mix the olive oil, eggs, buttermilk and vanilla extract together.

5   Now, make a well in the middle of the dry ingredients and pour in the wet ingredients and stir with a wooden spoon to combine. Don't overmix, as it should be a bit lumpy.

6   Divide the mixture evenly between the 12 paper cases and sprinkle the oats and sunflower seeds on top. Bake for 20 minutes until golden and a skewer inserted into the centre of the muffins comes out clean. Allow to cool in the tin for 5 minutes before turning out on to a wire rack to cool. Eat warm or cold.

Blueberry Muffins

Blueberry muffins are probably the most popular muffin flavour and they are incredibly easy to make. When making muffins it's very important not to overbeat the mixture, as it will exclude the precious air – the batter should be lumpy when you spoon it into the cases. Using low-fat, heart-healthy spread is an added bonus and any addition of fruit to a dessert will increase the nutritional benefit.

SERVE 12

250g (9oz) self-raising flour
1½ tsp baking powder
55g (2oz) low-fat, heart-healthy spread
85g (3oz) golden caster sugar
1 punnet blueberries (about 150g/5oz)
2 large eggs
235ml (8¼fl oz) skimmed milk
juice of ½ lemon

1 Preheat the oven to 180°C/350°F/Gas mark 4.

2 Line a 12-hole muffin tin with 12 paper muffin cases.

3 Sift the flour and baking powder into a large bowl. Add the low-fat spread and rub the spread into the flour gently with your fingertips until the mixture resembles breadcrumbs.

4 Now, stir in the sugar and blueberries and set aside.

5 Meanwhile, in another bowl, whisk the eggs, milk and lemon juice together. Add the egg mixture to the dry mixture and stir briefly. Try to do no more than 10 turns of your spoon. It should be combined but still lumpy.

6 Divide the mixture into the muffin cases and bake for 20–25 minutes or until a skewer inserted into the centre of the muffins comes out clean (apart from a little blueberry juice!). Allow to cool in the tin for 5 minutes, then transfer to a wire rack to cool. These muffins are delicious served warm.

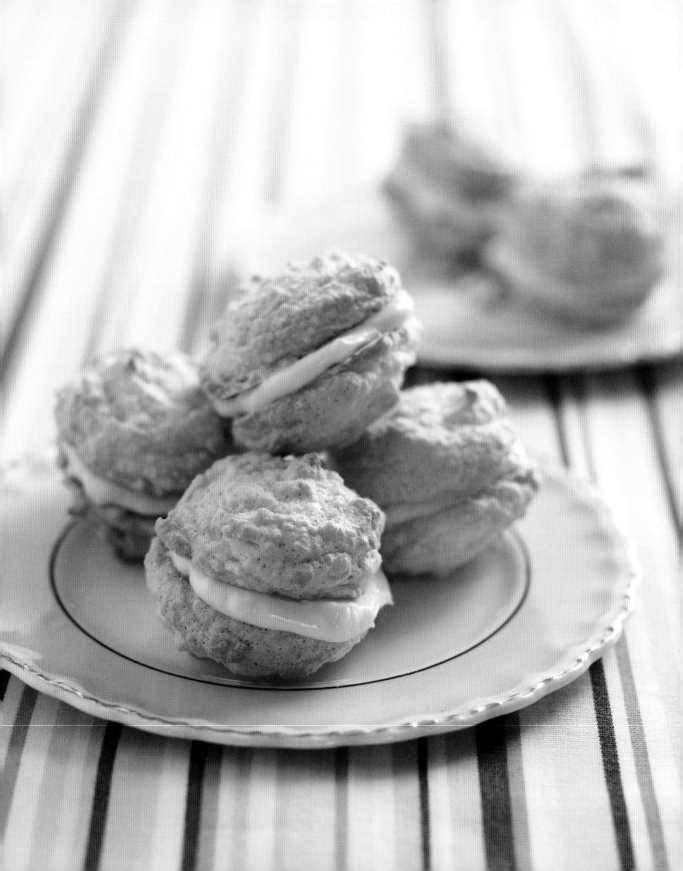

Almond Macaroons

Very low in fat, delicious and fun, these macaroons are so easy to make and you can even get the kids busy in the kitchen making these little morsels of deliciousness! You can colour the macaroons any shade you like, so get creative. I like to use natural food colouring to make blue, pink and, my personal favourite, purple macaroons. Simply add 3–4 drops of colour with the sugar.

MAKES 20

low-fat spread,
  for greasing (optional)
3 egg whites
150g (5½oz) caster sugar
2 drops vanilla extract
150g (5½oz) ground
  almonds
25g (1oz) plain flour,
  sifted
your choice of buttercream
  (see pages 182–183),
  optional

1   Preheat the oven to 180°C/350°F/Gas mark 4.

2   Either lightly grease a large non-stick baking tray with low-fat spread or line with non-stick baking parchment. If you don't have a large baking sheet, use numerous small ones.

3   In a large, very clean bowl, beat the egg whites until stiff peaks form. (An electric whisk is best, but if you want a good workout, do it by hand!) Continuing to whisk, gradually add the sugar until the egg whites are glossy and shiny.

4   Using a large, metal spoon, fold in the vanilla extract, ground almonds and sifted flour until combined.

5   Drop 2 teaspoons of the mixture into piles onto the prepared baking tray, leaving enough room to spread and bake for 15 minutes. Allow to cool on the baking tray for 5 minutes, then transfer the macaroons to a wire rack to cool. Eat just as they are or 'glued' together with a choice of buttercream.

Banana Chocolate Cupcakes

These days you can buy the most amazing paper cupcake cases, wonderful decorations and edible glitter. So go to town and pile these delicious, butter-free, cupcakes high!

MAKES 24

400g (14oz) caster sugar
245g (8¾oz) plain flour
75g (2½oz) good-quality
  cocoa powder
1½ tsp baking powder
½ tsp bicarbonate of soda
2 eggs
1 medium ripe banana,
  mashed
120ml (4fl oz) skimmed milk
120ml (4fl oz) vegetable oil
1½ tsp vanilla extract

For the low-fat
chocolate frosting
100g (3½oz) low-fat, heart-
  healthy spread, chilled
270g (9½oz) icing sugar,
  sifted
3 tbsp good-quality
  cocoa powder
skimmed milk,
  if required

To decorate
edible glitter
your choice of sprinkles

1 Preheat the oven to 180°C/350°F/Gas mark 4.

2 Line 2 x 12-hole muffin tins or a baking sheet with 24 paper muffin cases.

3 In a large bowl, mix the sugar, flour, cocoa powder, baking powder and bicarbonate of soda together.

4 In another large bowl, whisk the eggs, mashed banana, 240ml (8½fl oz) warm water, milk, vegetable oil and vanilla extract together.

5 Now, add the wet ingredients to the dry ingredients and stir, or whisk, until well combined.

6 Use an ice-cream scoop to transfer the mixture into the muffin cases until they are about three-quarters full and bake for about 20 minutes or until a cocktail stick inserted into the centre of a cupcake comes out clean. Leave in the tins or on the baking sheet for 5 minutes, then transfer to a wire rack to cool.

7 To make the frosting, simply put all the ingredients into a bowl and mix, either using a free-standing electric mixer or a hand whisk. An electric mixer gives a much better result because the sugar gets properly incorporated into the low-fat spread and gives a lovely, creamy and velvety texture.

recipe continues...

If you find that your banana
is not ripe enough to mash,
simply peel it and cook
in the microwave for
20 seconds. This will soften
the banana perfectly.

When filling muffin cases
with cake mixture, I find
that using an ice-cream
scoop usually makes the
job much easier and puts
in just the right amount
of mixture.

8 Put the frosting into the refrigerator for about
30 minutes before you pipe it, as the low-fat spread
can be much softer than butter and therefore more
difficult to pipe.

9 Use a piping bag fitted with a fluted nozzle to pipe the
frosting attractively on top of the cupcakes, then load
with as much edible glitter and sprinkles as you can!

Spicy Apple Muffins

Fat-free and deliciously spicy! With apple sauce replacing the butter and extra
added fibre, these spicy muffins will quickly become a healthy family favourite.

MAKES 16

175g (6oz) porridge oats
1 tsp bicarbonate of soda
2 tsp baking powder
1 tsp ground cinnamon
175g (6oz) wholemeal
  plain flour
4 egg whites, lightly
  beaten
470g (16½oz) homemade
  apple sauce
  (see page 185)
1 eating apple, peeled,
  cored and diced
150ml (5fl oz) clear,
  runny honey
125g (4½oz) low-fat
  crème fraîche

1 Preheat the oven to 180°C/350°F/Gas mark 4.

2 Put 16 paper muffins cases on a baking tray.

3 Sift all the dry ingredients into a large mixing bowl
and combine well.

4 Using a free-standing electric mixer, whisk the egg
whites until doubled in volume and stiff peaks form.

5 Now, add the apple sauce, diced apple, honey and
crème fraîche to the dry ingredients and stir together.
Using a large metal spoon or spatula, gently fold in
the whisked egg whites. Do not overmix.

6 Divide the mixture evenly between the 16 cases and
bake for 25 minutes or until lightly browned. Leave on
the baking tray for 5 minutes, then transfer to a wire
rack to cool. Eat warm or cold.

Breakfast in a Bun

These muffins include lots of healthy ingredients in just one mouthful to give you energy and to set you and yours up for a busy day. I make a batch of these when we are in the middle of a crazy few days – we all then just grab one as we pass by.

MAKES 12

300g (10½oz) wholemeal plain flour
50g (1¾oz) porridge oats
3 heaped tsp baking powder
½ tsp mixed spice
½ tsp ground cinnamon
150ml (5fl oz) low-fat buttermilk
150ml (5fl oz) skimmed milk
100ml (3½fl oz) light olive oil
1 medium egg, beaten
50g (1¾oz) soft brown sugar
grated zest of 1 lemon
2 tbsp lemon juice
2 small apples, washed, cored and grated
1 medium carrot, peeled and grated
100g (3½oz) raisins
50g (1¾oz) walnuts, chopped
100g (3½oz) ready-to-eat dried apricots, chopped
2 medium ripe bananas, peeled and mashed
sunflower and pumpkin seeds, for sprinkling

1 Preheat the oven to 190°C/375°F/Gas mark 5.

2 Line a 12-hole muffin tin with 12 large muffin cases.

3 Combine the flour, oats, baking powder and spices in a large bowl and set aside.

4 In another bowl, mix the buttermilk, milk, olive oil, egg and brown sugar together until combined.

5 Pour the wet ingredients into the dry ingredients and stir until just combined. Add the grated lemon zest and juice, grated apples, carrot, raisins, walnuts, apricots and mashed bananas and mix together but don't overmix.

6 Divide the mixture evenly between the muffin cases until they are three-quarters full, then sprinkle with the sunflower and pumpkin seeds. Bake for 20 minutes or until a skewer inserted into the centre comes out clean. Allow to cool in the tin for 5 minutes, then transfer the muffins to a wire rack to cool. Eat while still warm.

TIP
You can prepare the dry and wet ingredients the night before, then combine them in the morning. Pop the muffins into the oven and you'll have a freshly-baked breakfast.

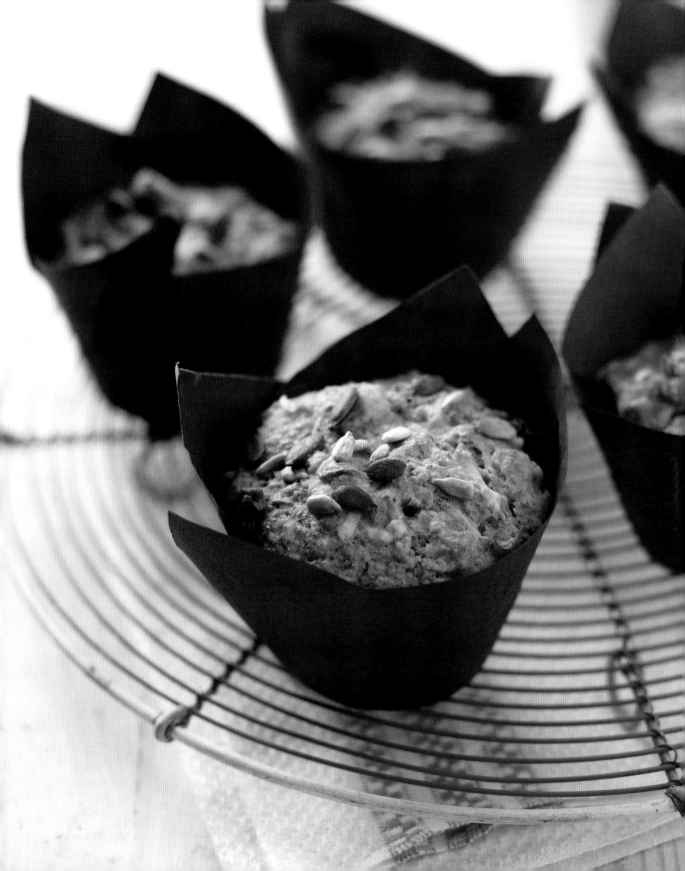

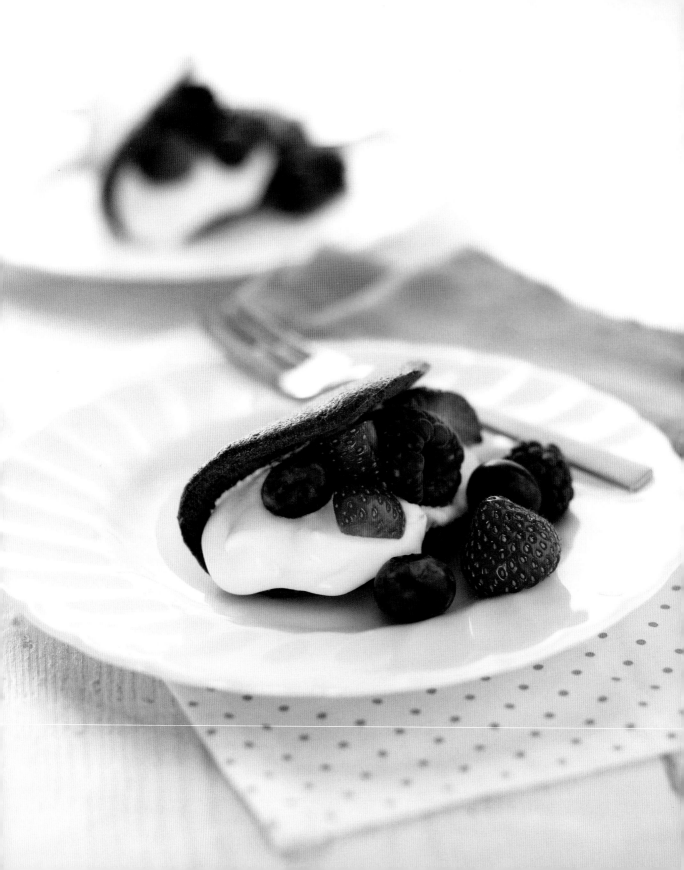

Chocolate Fruity Wraps

These light, fat-free chocolate sponges are wrapped around crème fraîche and a good helping of seasonal fruit. If you can't always buy good fresh fruit, canned is perfectly fine as long as it is in fruit juice and not syrup!

SERVES 8

2 eggs
4 tbsp caster sugar
6 tbsp plain flour
1½ tbsp cocoa powder

To serve
low-fat crème fraîche or
  fat-free Greek yogurt
any fruit you fancy, the
  more the better

1 Preheat the oven to 220°C/425°F/Gas mark 7.

2 Line 2 baking trays with greaseproof paper or a non-stick cooking sheet.

3 In a large bowl, whisk together the eggs and sugar until light and fluffy and the whisk leaves a trail when lifted from the mixture.

4 Next, sift the flour and cocoa into the egg mixture and fold in using a large, metal spoon. Don't overmix.

5 Now, drop rounded tablespoons of the mixture onto the prepared baking trays and spread them into oval shapes. Make sure they are spaced well apart as they will spread out during cooking. Bake for 6–8 minutes or until they are springy to the touch. Allow to cool on the baking trays.

6 When they are nearly cool, gently fold in half without splitting the sponges and leave until completely cold. To serve, fill with low-fat crème fraîche or Greek yogurt and lots of fruit.

Healthy Scones

For some reason my children perceive scones to be 'caring'! Maybe it's because if one of them is upset or struggling, my usual answer is to make them a plate of scones and a cup of warm milk. Give it a go – it might make you feel better too.

SERVES 10-14

light cooking oil spray,
  for coating
165g (5½oz) wholemeal
  flour
140g (5oz) plain flour
2 tsp baking powder
½ tsp bicarbonate of soda
55g (2oz) low-fat, heart-
  healthy spread, chilled
150g (5½oz) homemade
  apple sauce (see
  page 185)
75ml (3fl oz) low-fat
  buttermilk
50g (1¾oz) raisins
a splash of skimmed milk,
  for brushing

TIP
Pop the low-fat spread in the freezer for 10 minutes before using, otherwise it may be a little too soft.

1 Preheat the oven to 200°C/400°F/Gas mark 6.

2 Spray a baking sheet with cooking oil spray.

3 In a large bowl, combine all the flours, baking powder and bicarbonate of soda.

4 Add the chilled, low-fat spread to the flour and, using a knife, cut into the flour. Rub the spread into the flour with your fingertips until the mixture resembles breadcrumbs.

5 Now, stir in the apple sauce and just enough of the buttermilk to form a stiff dough. Fold in the raisins and form into a ball of dough. Turn out onto a lightly floured surface and roll out the dough until it is about 1.5 cm (⅝in) thick. Use a cookie cutter to cut out the scones and place onto the prepared baking tray.

6 Brush the tops of the scones with the milk and bake for 16–18 minutes or until lightly browned, then transfer to a wire rack to cool. Delicious eaten warm or cool.

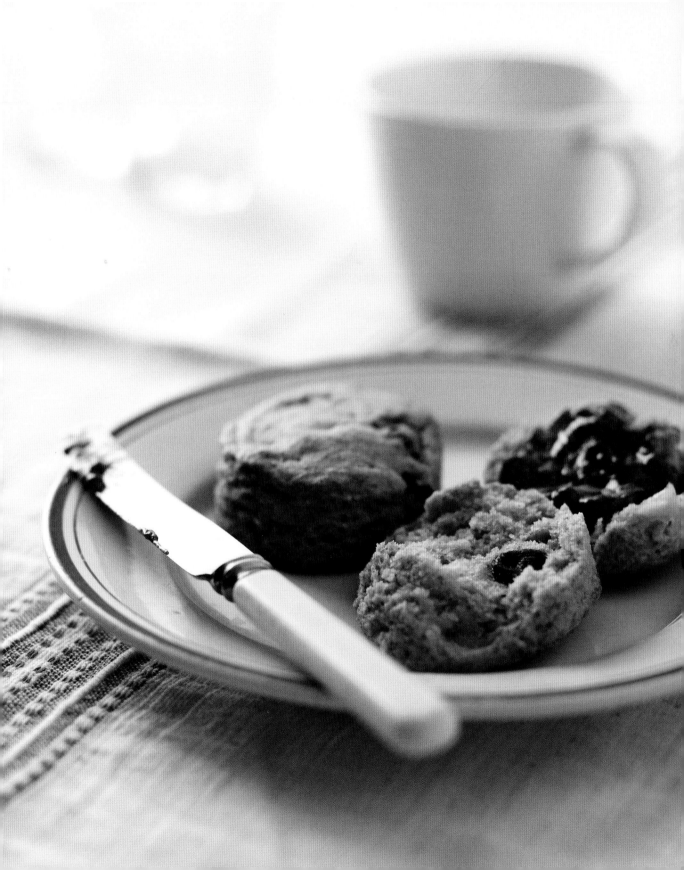

High Fibre Muffins

These healthy little treats offer you a great high fibre content and are low in saturated fat. Perfect! They are lovely eaten either warm or cold.

MAKES 12

140g (5oz) high fibre
  bran cereal
  (the one that looks like
  little matchsticks!)
250ml (9 fl oz) skimmed
  milk
140g (5oz) plain flour
1 tbsp baking powder
1 tsp ground cinnamon
½ tsp ground nutmeg
½ tsp ground ginger
  (optional)
115g (4oz) soft light
  brown sugar
100g (3½oz) raisins
2 eggs
6 tbsp sunflower oil

1 Preheat the oven to 200°C/400°F/Gas mark 6.

2 Line a 12-hole muffin tin with paper cases.

3 Put the cereal in a bowl with the skimmed milk and leave to soak for 5 minutes until the cereal has softened. Set aside.

4 Sift the flour, baking powder, cinnamon, nutmeg and ginger (if using) together into a large bowl, then stir in the sugar and raisins.

5 In a separate jug, beat together the eggs and the sunflower oil. Make a well in the middle of the dry ingredients and pour in the egg mixture and the cereal and milk and combine all the ingredients gently. Don't overmix, as it should be a bit lumpy.

6 Spoon the mixture into the paper cases and bake for 20 minutes or until well risen and golden. Allow to cool in the tin for 5 minutes before turning out onto a wire rack to cool.

Honey & Parsnip Scones

Parsnips have useful amounts of vitamin C, vitamin E and potassium, while the low-fat spread makes these scones lower in fat than others, so they make a fabulous alternative scone.

MAKES 10-14

550g (1lb 4oz) parsnips, peeled and cut into 2.5cm (1in) cubes
55g (2oz) low-fat, heart-healthy spread, chilled
900g (2lb) self-raising flour
½ teaspoon English mustard powder (optional)
5 tsp clear, runny honey
4 eggs
a splash of skimmed milk
1 egg yolk, beaten, for brushing
plain flour, for dusting

TIP
Pop the low-fat, heart-healthy spread in the freezer for 10 minutes before using, otherwise it may be too soft.

1 Preheat the oven to 190°C/375°F/Gas mark 5.

2 Line 2 baking sheets with non-stick baking parchment.

3 Boil the parsnips for about 15 minutes or until tender. Drain and dip into a bowl of cold water. Set aside.

4 In a large bowl, rub the chilled low-fat spread, flour and mustard powder together with your fingertips until the mixture resembles breadcrumbs.

5 Now, mash the parsnips roughly, leaving them quite chunky and stir into the flour mixture.

6 Next, stir in the honey and eggs and slowly add enough milk to form a soft pliable dough. Using floured hands, form into a ball of dough, then remove from the bowl and knead lightly on a floured surface until the dough is smooth and elastic. Roll the dough out to about 2.5cm (1in) thick, then cut into rounds using a cookie cutter and place on the prepared baking sheets.

7 Brush the tops of the scones with a little beaten egg yolk and bake for 15–20 minutes or until golden brown on top and hollow when tapped on the base. Transfer to a wire rack to cool. Delicious eaten warm or cool.

Raspberry Muffins

Muffins are a great low-fat option for cakes. Feel free to have a play and add other fruits, nuts or chocolate chips if you are really treating yourself. White chocolate goes beautifully with raspberries – but not everytime!

MAKES 12

250g (9oz) self-raising flour
1½ tsp baking powder
55g (2oz) low-fat, heart-
   healthy spread, chilled
85g (3oz) caster sugar
1 punnet raspberries,
   washed (about
   200g/7oz)
2 large eggs
235ml (8¼fl oz) skimmed
   milk
juice of ½ lemon

1 Preheat the oven to 180°C/350°F/Gas mark 4.

2 Line a 12-hole muffin tin with paper muffin cases.

3 Sift the flour and baking powder into a large bowl. Add the low-fat spread and rub it into the flour gently with your fingertips until the mixture resembles breadcrumbs.

4 Now, stir in the sugar, then add the berries and stir very carefully.

5 In a separate bowl, whisk the eggs, milk and lemon juice together using a fork or hand whisk. Add this to the dry mixture and stir briefly (enough to combine the mixture but leaving it lumpy and taking care of the raspberries).

6 Dollop the mixture evenly into the paper cases and bake for 20–25 minutes. Eat warm – delicious!

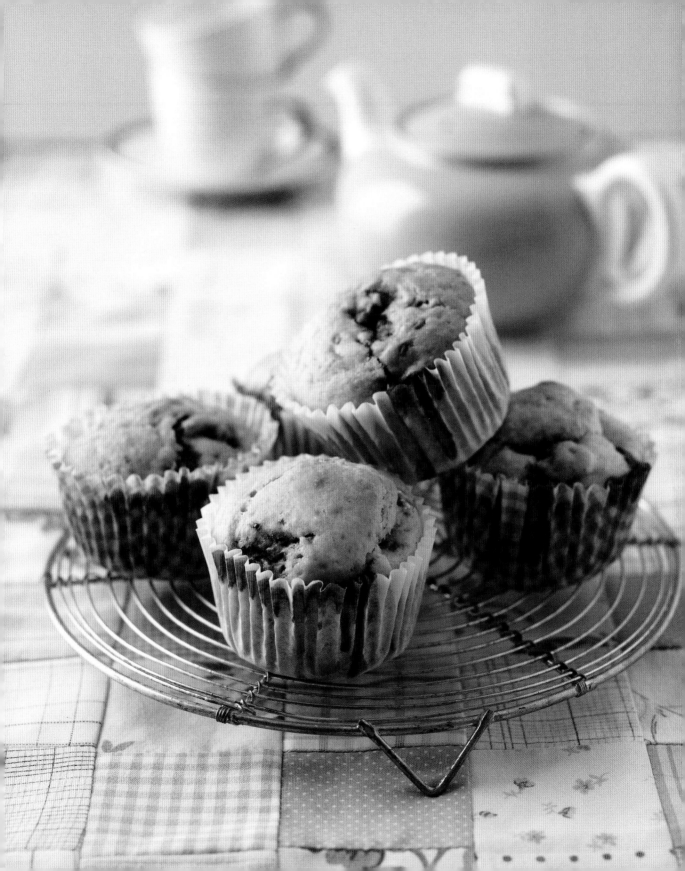

Gluten-free Chocolate Whoopies

This recipe was kindly donated to me by Sophie Grey, a gluten-free expert! Sophie says, 'I was asked to develop this recipe for the *Black Swan* film premiere. They looked absolutely magnificent and so elegant.'

MAKES 15
MEDIUM WHOOPIES,
ABOUT 4–5CM (1½–2IN)

140g (5oz) soya flour
30g (1oz) cocoa powder
1 tsp bicarbonate of soda
100ml (3½fl oz) buttermilk
100ml (3½fl oz) milk
1 tsp vanilla extract
80g (3oz) unsalted butter
100g (3½oz) demerara
  sugar
1 egg, beaten

For the filling
50g (1¾oz) butter
100g (3½oz) icing sugar
150g (5½oz) cream cheese
1 tsp vanilla extract

1   Preheat the oven to 200°C/400°F/Gas mark 6.

2   Line a baking tray with non-stick baking parchment.

3   Sift the dry ingredients together. Put the buttermilk, milk and vanilla extract into another bowl and set aside.

4   Cream the butter and demerara sugar together with a hand-held electric whisk, a free-standing mixer using the whisk attachment or a hand-held balloon whisk if you have the energy, until the butter and sugar mixture is pale and fluffy.

5   Once the mixture is pale, slowly add the beaten egg while continuing to whisk.

6   Once the egg has been incorporated, alternately fold the wet ingredients into the dry ingredients with a large metal spoon using a figure-of-eight action, keeping the air in the mixture. Mix until it is an even colour, but do not overmix.

recipe continues...

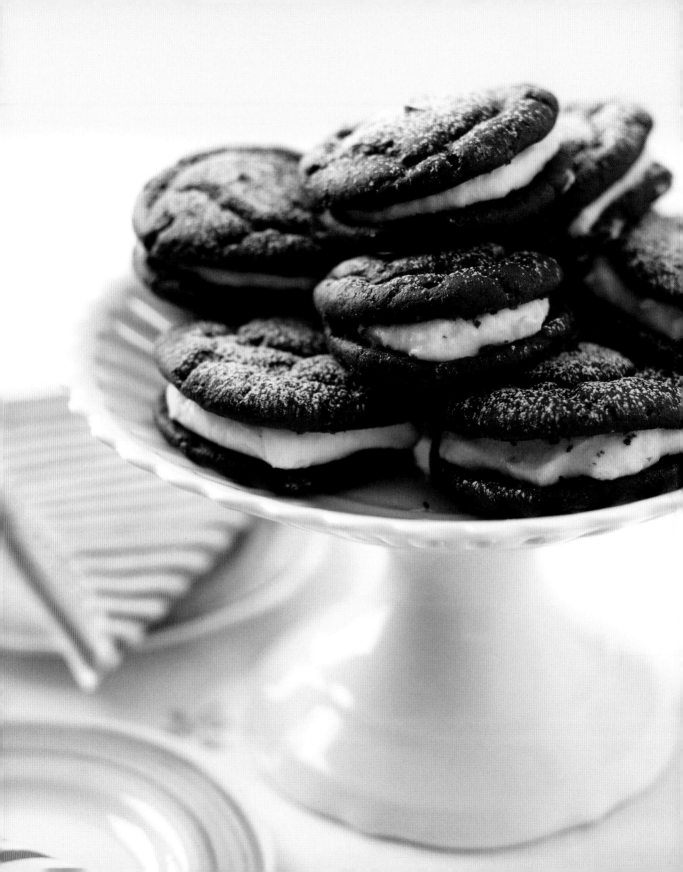

7 Pipe or use a dessertspoon to spoon 30 x 3cm (1¼in) dollops onto the prepared baking tray, making sure the dollops are at least 3cm (1¼in) high and spaced well apart to allow for spreading during cooking. Bake for 6–8 minutes or until firm to the touch. To check, slightly open the oven and touch the top of the nearest whoopee to you. Either allow to cool on the baking tray or transfer to a wire rack to cool.

8 To make the filling, cream the butter and icing sugar together in a bowl. Add the cream cheese and vanilla extract and mix until smooth, but don't overmix.

9 Once the whoopies are cooled, sandwich together two whoopie halves with the cream cheese filling and serve.

BREADS

Courgette & Cranberry Loaf

This loaf is so incredibly easy and is perfect to have on hand to fill in the gaps. Served just warm or cold, it's perfect either way.

MAKES 2 LOAVES

225ml (8fl oz) light olive oil, plus extra for oiling
425g (15oz) plain flour
400g (14oz) granulated sugar
1 tsp ground cinnamon
1 tsp ground nutmeg
a pinch of Maldon sea salt
1 tsp bicarbonate of soda
½ tsp baking powder
3 eggs
300g (10½oz) shredded courgette
75g (3oz) chopped walnuts or pecan nuts
100g (3½oz) halved fresh or frozen cranberries

1 Preheat the oven to 180°C/350°F/gas mark 4.

2 Oil two 23 x 12cm (9 x 5in) loaf tins with a little olive oil.

3 In a large bowl, combine all the dry ingredients together.

4 In another bowl, mix the eggs, olive oil and shredded courgette together, then add to the flour mixture and, using a wooden spoon, mix until combined but still a little lumpy.

5 Now, add the nuts and finally the cranberries, being careful not to break them up too much.

6 Divide the mixture between the prepared loaf tins and bake for 50–60 minutes or until a skewer inserted into the centre of each loaf comes out clean. Allow to cool in the tins for 10 minutes before turning out onto a wire rack to cool. Delicious eaten warm or cold.

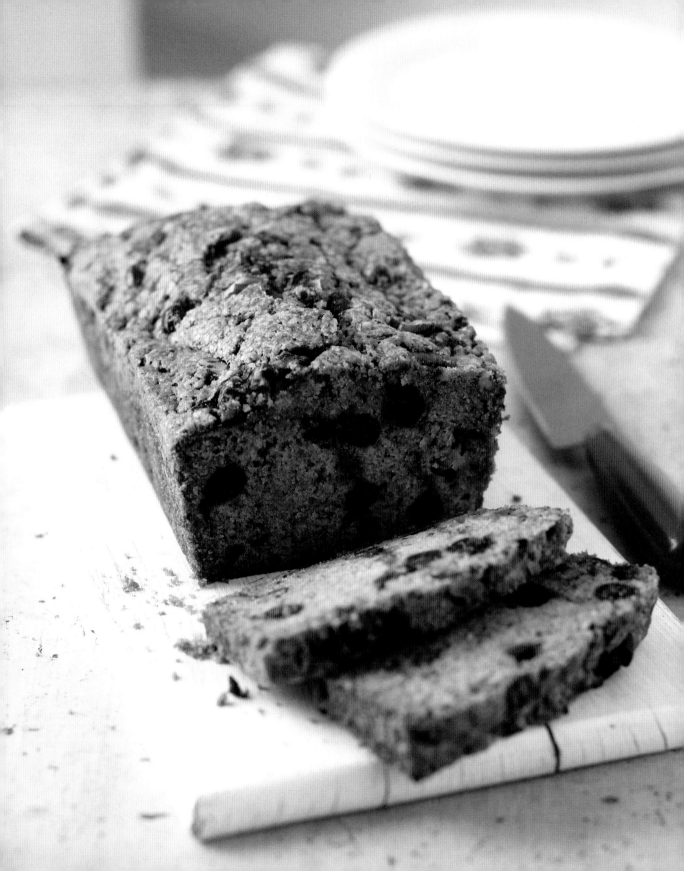

Oatmeal Fruit Bread

I make a batch of this when we are planning a picnic with friends – and usually the friends we are meeting end up eating more of our food than their own! How can that be right?

MAKES 1 LOAF

light cooking oil spray,
   for coating
425g (15oz) can pears in
   natural juice, drained
200g (7oz) wholemeal
   plain flour
45g (1½oz) porridge oats
100g (3½oz) dark brown
   sugar
1 tsp baking powder
½ tsp bicarbonate of soda
1 large egg, beaten
3 tbsp vegetable oil
25g (1oz) oatbran
90g (3¼oz) chopped dried
   fruit, such as apricots,
   prunes, dates, raisins,
   dried cranberries
   or dried blueberries
75g (3oz) chopped walnuts
   or pecan nuts

TIP
I prefer to eat this loaf
the next day. Wrap in a
large sheet of greaseproof
paper and store overnight
before slicing.

1   Preheat the oven to 170°C/325°F/Gas mark 3.

2   Spray a 23 x 12cm (9 x 5in) loaf tin with cooking oil spray.

3   Drain the pears, reserving the juice, then place the pears in a blender and process until smooth.

4   Pour the puréed pears into a measuring jug and top up with the reserved juice to make a volume of 310ml (just over 10fl oz).

5   Put the flour, oats, sugar, baking powder and bicarbonate of soda in a large bowl and stir to mix, pressing out any lumps in the brown sugar with the back of the spoon. Set aside.

6   Now, add the beaten egg and vegetable oil to the pears and stir to mix, then add the pear mixture to the flour mixture and stir until combined.

7   Finally, add the oatbran, dried fruit and nuts to the mixture and stir to mix. Pour the mixture into the prepared loaf tin and bake for about 45 minutes or until a skewer inserted into the centre of the loaf comes out clean.

8   Remove the bread from the oven, leave in the tin for 10 minutes, then turn out onto a wire rack until to cool completely. Eat warm or cold.

Olive Bread

Shop-bought bread can be very high in salt and speciality breads can be expensive. All my bread recipes are low in salt, easy to make and inexpensive. So, even if you've never made bread before, you'll be sure to succeed. Buy good-quality olives to make the most of this Mediterranean inspired bread.

MAKES 1 LOAF

1 tsp caster sugar
3 tsp dried active yeast
700g (1½lb) wholemeal
  flour, plus extra for dusting
a pinch of Maldon sea salt
60ml (2fl oz) extra virgin
  olive oil, plus extra for
  sprinkling and oiling
175g (6oz) good-quality
  black olives, pitted and
  cut into quarters

1   Pour 60ml (2fl oz) warm water into a bowl. Mix in the sugar, then sprinkle the yeast on top and set aside to ferment and bubble for about 5 minutes.

2   Put the flour into a large bowl and add the yeast mixture and a pinch of salt. Add 350ml (12fl oz) hand-hot water and begin mixing together with a wooden spoon.

3   Next, add the olive oil and mix again. You may need to use your hands at this point.

4   Turn the dough out onto a lightly floured surface and knead for 10 minutes, then add the quartered olives.

5   Place the dough in a bowl with a sprinkling of olive oil on top, cover with a damp cloth and leave in a warm place for about 1½ hours. By this time the dough should have doubled in size.

6   Once risen, put the dough on a baking sheet without kneading but tugging the sides underneath all the way around repeatedly for about 3 minutes. Cover with a clean, damp tea towel and let the dough rise again in a warm place for about 1 hour or until doubled in size.

recipe continues...

7   Preheat the oven to 230°C/450°F/Gas mark 8 and oil a baking tray with a little olive oil.

8   When the bread has doubled in size again, place on the prepared baking tray and bake for 20 minutes. Lower the oven temperature to 190°C/375°F/Gas mark 5 and bake for a further 20 minutes. If the bread sounds hollow when you tap the base, it is cooked. If it doesn't, bake for 5 more minutes. Transfer to a wire rack to cool. Eat warm or cold.

Soda Bread

I love to have soda bread when I'm in Ireland – it's a tasty and lighter alternative to standard bread. Try this version and serve with boiled eggs and, as the Irish would say, 'a cup o' tea'!

MAKES 1 LOAF

170g (6oz) plain flour, plus extra for dusting
170g (6oz) wholemeal self-raising flour
½ tsp Maldon sea salt
½ tsp bicarbonate of soda
290ml (10fl oz) low-fat buttermilk

1   Preheat the oven to 200°C/400°F/Gas mark 6 and lightly dust a baking sheet with flour.

2   Place the flours, salt and bicarbonate of soda into a large mixing bowl and stir together to combine.

3   Make a well in the centre, pour in the buttermilk and mix with a large fork to form a soft dough.

4   Turn the dough onto a lightly floured surface and knead for about 5 minutes.

5   Shape into a round and flatten the dough slightly before placing on the prepared baking sheet.

6   Cut a cross on the top and bake for about 30 minutes or until the loaf sounds hollow when tapped on the base. Allow to cool on a wire rack and serve warm. Yum!

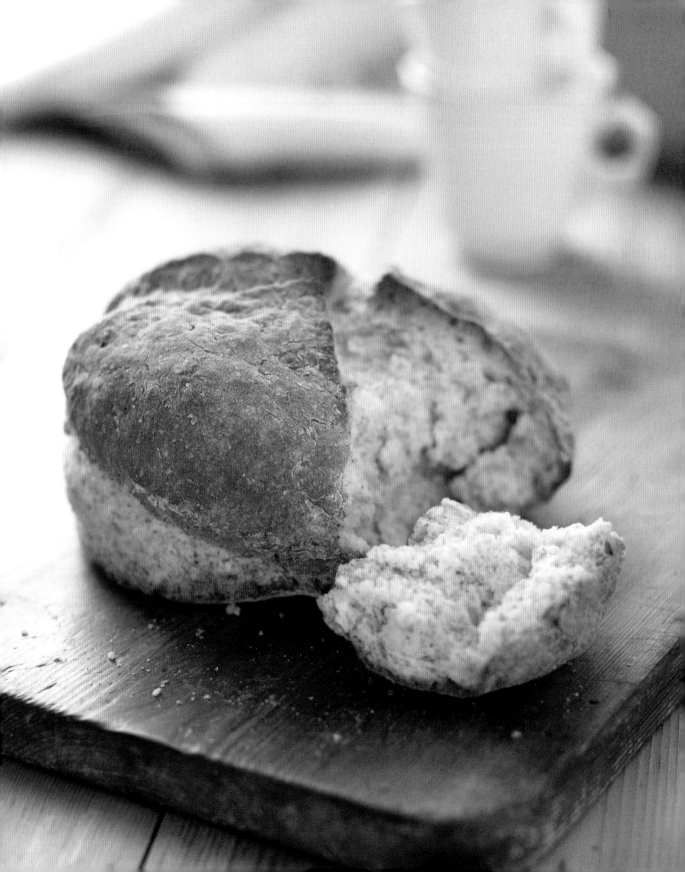

Onion Focaccia Bread

Focaccia bread is easier than you might think and nothing beats the flavour when freshly baked. As a special treat, this bread works well with a little low-fat mozzarella grilled on the top after the bread has been baked in the oven.

MAKES 1 LOAF

3 tbsp olive oil,
  plus extra for oiling
300g (10½oz) plain flour,
  plus extra for dusting
½ tsp Maldon sea salt,
  plus extra for sprinkling
1 x 7g (¼oz) packet easy-
  blend dried yeast
1 tbsp chopped
  fresh rosemary
1 tbsp chopped
  fresh sage leaves
2 tsp chopped,
  fresh parsley,
1 small onion, peeled
  and finely sliced

1 Oil a baking sheet and a piece of clingfilm with a little olive oil.

2 Sift the flour and salt into a large bowl and stir in the dried yeast and chopped herbs.

3 Pour in 2 tablespoons of olive oil and 250ml (9fl oz) warm water and mix with your hands until a soft dough forms.

4 Turn the dough out onto a lightly floured surface and knead for about 5 minutes until the dough is smooth and elastic.

5 Place the dough onto the prepared baking tray and press out with your knuckles to make a 24cm (9½in) rough shaped round. Cover with the oiled clingfilm and leave in a warm place for about 1 hour or until doubled in size.

6 Preheat the oven to 220°C/425°F/Gas mark 7.

7 Now, remove the clingfilm and sprinkle the dough with the sliced onion and a little salt and drizzle the remaining olive oil over the top.

8 Bake in the oven for about 25 minutes. Check that the bread is cooked by tapping it on the base – if it sounds hollow, it's done. If not, put it back in the oven for another 5 minutes. Turn out onto a wire rack to cool. Eat warm or cold.

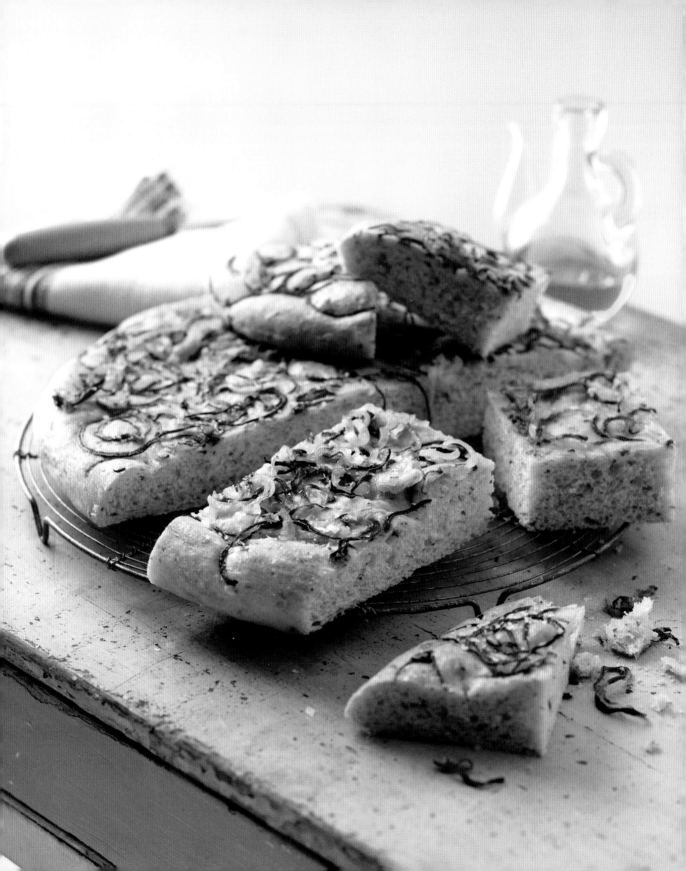

Rustic Nutty Spring Onion Loaf

Don't be afraid to be inventive with your bread recipes. The hazelnuts and walnuts in this loaf make it different and incredibly nutty!

MAKES 1 LOAF

olive oil, for oiling
450g (1lb) wholemeal flour, plus extra for dusting
1 tsp Maldon sea salt
25g (1oz) chopped hazelnuts
25g (1oz) chopped walnuts
100g (3½oz) mixed seeds (such as poppy seeds, pumpkin seeds and sunflower seeds)
1 tbsp clear, runny honey
1 x 7g (¼oz) packet easy-blend dried yeast
6 spring onions, washed and sliced

1   Oil a baking tray with a little olive oil.

2   Put the flour, salt, nuts and seeds into a large bowl and mix together.

3   Pour 300ml (10fl oz) warm water into another bowl and add the honey and yeast. Mix together and set aside for 5 minutes.

4   Make a well in the centre of the flour mixture, add the liquid and spring onions, and work together with your hands to form a ball of dough.

5   Turn the dough onto a lightly floured surface and knead well for at least 5 minutes.

6   Pop the dough into a bowl, cover with a clean, damp tea towel and leave in a warm place for 2 hours until the dough has doubled in size.

7   Knead the dough energetically again on a lightly floured surface for 5 minutes, then put onto an oiled baking sheet, cover again with a damp tea towel and leave in a warm place for another hour.

8   Preheat the oven to 220°C/425°F/gas mark 7.

9   Now, bake the bread for 30–35 minutes. Check that the bread is cooked by tapping it on the base; if it sounds hollow, it's done. If not, put it back in the oven for another 5 minutes. Serve warm or cold.

Rye Bread

Rye bread is heavier and therefore will keep you feeling fuller for longer. It also keeps well and makes a perfect packed lunch. Slice thinly and eat plain or with just a small amount of low-fat, heart-healthy spread.

MAKES 1 LOAF

30g (1oz) easy-blend
  dried yeast
300g (10½oz) rye flour
200g (7oz) strong plain
  bread flour, plus extra
  for dusting
1 tsp Maldon sea salt
3 tbsp linseeds
2 tbsp poppy seeds
2 tbsp sesame seeds
3 tbsp sunflower seeds
olive oil, for oiling
300g (10½oz) porridge
  oats

1 Stir the dried yeast into 255ml (9fl oz) warm water and set aside for 5 minutes.

2 In a large mixing bowl, combine the rye flour, strong flour, salt, linseeds, poppy seeds, sesame seeds and sunflower seeds.

3 Make a well in the centre, add the yeast mixture and mix together with your hands until it becomes a soft, pliable dough. Place the dough onto a clean, lightly floured surface and knead for 5 minutes.

4 Return the dough to the bowl, cover with a damp, clean tea towel and leave in a warm place for an hour to rise. There is no need to knead the dough for a second time.

5 Preheat the oven to 200°C/400°F/Gas mark 6 and oil a baking tray with a little olive oil.

6 Now, shape the dough into a loaf shape, and roll the loaf in the oats. With a sharp knife, cut a line down the centre of the loaf and place on the prepared baking sheet.

7 Bake for 30 minutes or until golden brown and it sounds hollow when tapped on the base. Transfer the loaf to a wire rack and allow to cool for at least 30 minutes before slicing.

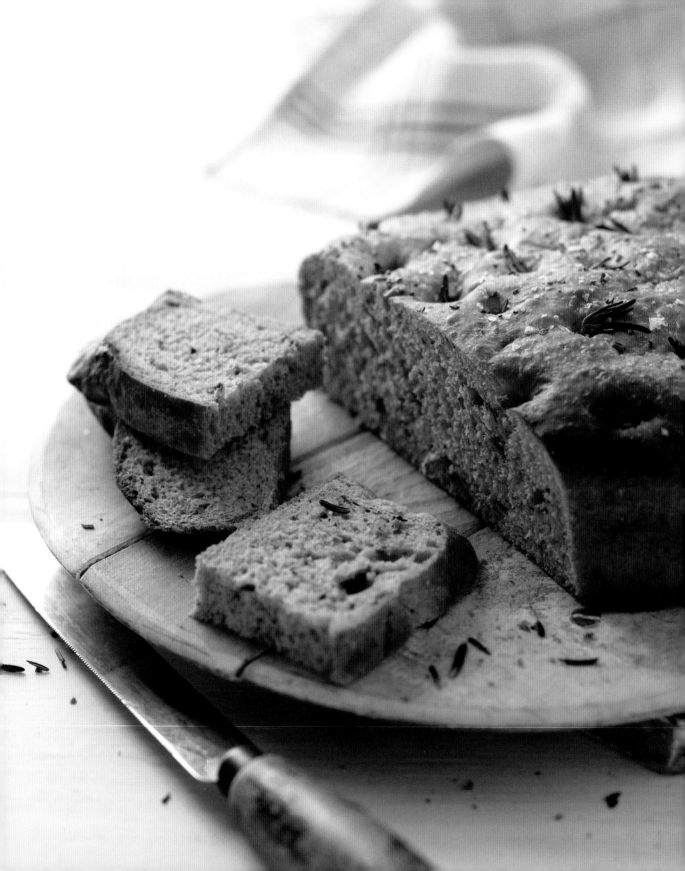

Sun-dried Tomato Bread

Packed with flavour from the sun-dried tomatoes, which you can either buy ready prepared or make yourself! Tomatoes are good for you however they are prepared and this loaf gives you the best of both flavour and goodness.

MAKES 1 LOAF

light cooking spray or
    olive oil, for coating
425g (15oz) strong white
    bread flour, plus extra
    for dusting
1 tsp Maldon sea salt,
    plus extra for sprinkling
50g (1¾oz) sun-dried
    tomatoes, chopped and
    drained (reserve the oil)
3 tbsp sun-dried tomato
    paste
2 tbsp chopped oregano
    or rosemary, plus finely
    chopped herbs,
    for sprinkling
1 x 7g (¼oz) packet easy-
    blend dried yeast
fresh rosemary sprigs

1   Spray a 23cm (9in) round cake tin with light cooking spray or olive oil.

2   Put the flour, salt, sun-dried tomatoes and paste into a large bowl. Add the chopped herbs and yeast, then pour in 325ml (11fl oz) warm water. Mix together with your hands until the mixture combines to make a rough ball of dough. Tip the dough out onto a lightly floured surface and stretch and knead the dough for 10 minutes until smooth and elastic.

3   Put the dough into the prepared tin and, using your finger, press lots of indentations into the top of the bread. Insert a small rosemary stalk into each hole and scatter over a few extra chopped herbs, then drizzle with some of the reserved oil from the sun-dried tomatoes and sprinkle with a little extra salt.

4   Cover loosely with clingfilm and leave in a warm place for 30–40 minutes until doubled in size.

5   Preheat the oven to 200°C/400°F/Gas mark 6.

6   Remove the clingfilm and bake the bread for 35 minutes until golden. Transfer to a wire rack to cool. Serve warm or cold. Just be careful, as the tomatoes will be very hot straight out of the oven.

Three-Seed Rolls

These seeded rolls look absolutely gorgeous – and they don't taste half bad too. They are very easy to make and have a slightly sweet edge, but my problem is that one just isn't enough!

MAKES 12 ROLLS

3 tsp sunflower oil, plus
  extra for oiling
1 x 7g (¼oz) packet easy-
  blend dried yeast
3 tsp golden syrup
¼ tsp Maldon sea salt
350g (12oz) wholemeal
  flour, plus extra for dusting
55g (2oz) sunflower seeds
55g (2oz) sesame seeds
55g (2oz) pumpkin seeds

1 Oil a baking sheet with a little sunflower oil.

2 Mix the yeast with a teaspoon of golden syrup and 200ml (7fl oz) warm water. Leave to stand for about 10 minutes until frothy.

3 Pour the rest of the syrup, the salt, oil and flour into a large mixing bowl. Pour the yeast mixture into the flour and knead together to form a ball of dough.

4 Put the dough on a clean, lightly floured surface and knead well for 5 minutes.

5 Now, oil a bowl with a little extra sunflower oil. Transfer the dough to the bowl, cover with a clean, damp tea towel and leave to rest in a warm place for about an hour or until it has doubled in size.

6 Take the dough out of the bowl and push the dough down to knock out the air. Now, add the seeds and knead until the seeds are incorporates into the dough. Continue to knead well for about 5 minutes.

7 Divide the dough up into 12 equal portions and roll each into a ball. Place on the prepared baking sheet, cover again with a clean, damp tea towel and leave in a warm place for at least another 40 minutes. Longer would be good.

8 Preheat the oven to 210°C/415°F/Gas mark 6-7.

9 Bake the rolls for 20–25 minutes. To check if the rolls are cooked, turn over and tap the base. If they sound hollow, they are cooked. If not, cook for a further 3 minutes. Transfer to a wire rack. Best eaten warm!

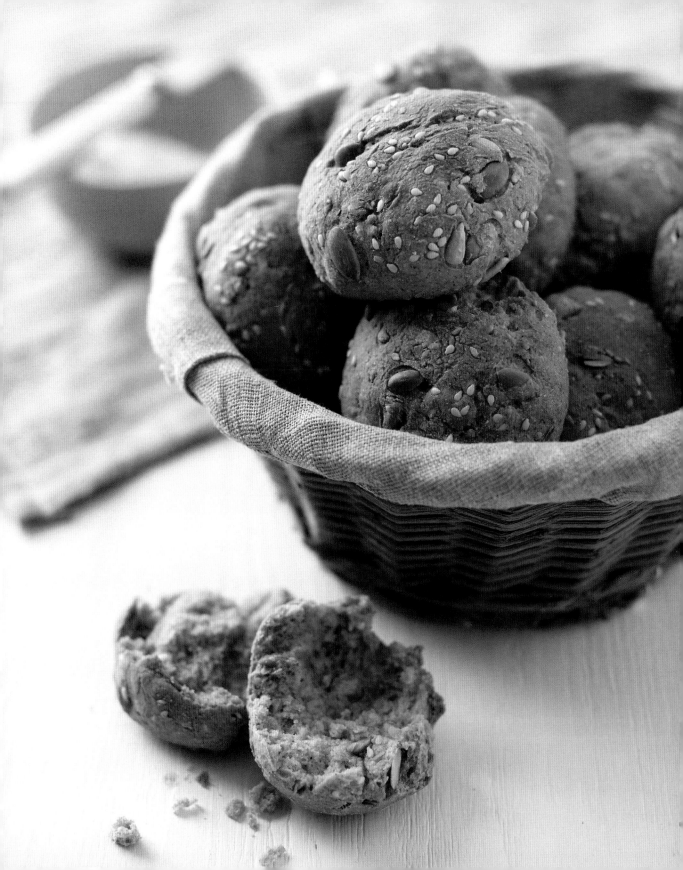

Wholemeal Herby Onion Bread

This is one of my favourite recipes and I probably make a loaf of this once a week. The herbs and onion give the bread a distinctive taste that is just a bit too more-ish.

MAKES 1 LOAF

1 x 7g (¼oz) packet
  easy-blend dried yeast
700g (1½lb) strong
  wholemeal flour,
  plus extra for dusting
2 tsp Maldon sea salt
1 large onion, peeled,
  sliced and very
  finely chopped
1 tbsp chopped parsley
1 tbsp chopped thyme
1 tbsp chopped sage
1 tbsp olive oil, plus
  extra for oiling
1 tbsp sesame seeds
  (optional)

1 Start by mixing the yeast with 200ml (7fl oz) warm water and set aside for about 10 minutes until frothy.

2 In a large bowl, mix the flour and salt together.

3 Make a well into the flour and add the yeast mixture, 200ml (7fl oz) warm water, chopped onion, herbs and olive oil and mix to a dough.

4 Turn the dough out onto a lightly floured surface and knead energetically for 10 minutes until the dough is smooth and elastic.

5 Oil a bowl and a baking sheet with a little olive oil. Put the dough into the bowl, cover with a clean, damp tea towel and leave to rise in a warm place for about 1 hour or until doubled in size.

6 Preheat the oven to 220°C/425°F/Gas mark 7.

7 Turn the dough onto a floured surface, knock back with your hand or fist to remove any air pockets and knead again for just a few minutes. Pop a baking tray in the oven for 5 minutes to warm, then remove from the oven and oil with a little olive oil.

recipe continues...

8   Form the dough into a smooth ball and place on the oiled baking tray. Brush with water and sprinkle on the sesame seeds (if using). Cover and leave in a warm place for about 30 minutes or until it has almost doubled in size.

9   Bake for 20 minutes, then lower the temperature to 190°C/375°F/Gas Mark 5 and continue to bake for a further 15–20 minutes or until the bread sounds hollow when tapped on the base. Turn out onto a wire rack to cool and enjoy warm or cold.

Wholemeal Pitta Bread

I counsel heart patients and one of the problems that many seem to face is insomnia. This is such a debilitating condition that can very quickly get out of hand. If you are struggling to drop off to sleep at night, I often recommend a slice of wholemeal pitta bread with a dollop of low-fat hummous. It gives just the right amount of carbohydrate to tire you out but not too much that it keeps you awake!

MAKES 8

2 tsp easy-blend
  dried yeast
1 tsp caster sugar
310ml (just over 10fl oz)
  warm skimmed milk
635g (1lb 6oz) wholemeal
  flour, plus extra
  for dusting
1 tsp Maldon sea salt
125ml (4fl oz) low-fat
  plain yogurt
1 egg, beaten
1 tbsp light olive oil,
  plus extra for oiling

1   Combine the yeast, sugar and milk in a small bowl and whisk until the yeast is dissolved. Cover the bowl and leave to stand in a warm place for 10 minutes or until the mixture is frothy.

2   Sift the flour and salt into a large bowl, mix and make a well in the middle. Pour in the yeast mixture with the yogurt, beaten egg, 60ml (2fl oz) warm water and olive oil and work this into the flour to form a ball of dough.

   recipe continues...

3 Turn the dough out onto a lightly floured surface and knead for 10 minutes until the dough is smooth and elastic.

4 Oil a bowl with a little olive oil and put the dough into the bowl. Cover and leave in a warm place for about an hour or until doubled in size.

5 Turn the dough out onto a floured surface and knead until very smooth. Divide the dough up into 8 portions and knead each portion into a ball.

6 Lightly flour a baking tray . Place the dough balls on the prepared tray, cover with a dry tea towel and leave in a warm place for 30 minutes or until well risen.

7 Preheat the oven to the highest temperature.

8 Now, on a lightly floured surface and using a rolling pin, roll each ball down into a 25cm (10in) round or oval.

9 Heat the baking tray in the very hot oven for 5 minutes, then cook one or two pittas at a time, depending on how big your tray is. Bake for just 5 minutes or until the bread is nicely browned and beginning to expand. Once cooked, wrap the cooked pittas in a dry clean cloth to keep warm before serving.

COOKIES

Ginger Biscuits

This is a really simple recipe for an old-fashioned favourite. You'll never need to buy a packet of ginger biscuits again. Here, low-fat, heart-healthy spread replaces the butter making them a healthier alternative to shop-bought biscuits.

MAKES 16

125g (4½oz) low-fat, heart-healthy spread
125g (4½oz) demerara sugar
1 egg yolk
1 tbsp golden syrup
180g (6¼oz) self-raising flour
1 tsp ground ginger
plain flour, for dusting

1   Preheat the oven to 180°C/350°F/Gas mark 4.

2   Line 2 baking sheets with non-stick baking parchment.

3   Beat the low-fat spread and sugar together in a bowl until smooth and creamy using a wooden spoon.

4   Add the egg yolk and golden syrup and mix together thoroughly.

5   Now, sift the flour and ground ginger into the mixture and gently mix. If the mixture is a little too dry, add a tiny bit of water.

6   Next, using dry hands, work the biscuit dough into a ball. If you keep the dough moving in your hands, it shouldn't stick too much. Once you have control of the dough, put it onto a lightly floured surface.

7   Divide the mixture into 16 small balls if you want small biscuits or, of course, you can make 8 jumbo sized ones if you choose! Roll each ball in the palm of your hand and place onto the prepared baking trays, squashing each down flat with the palm of your hand. Leave space between each one, as they will spread during cooking.

8   Bake for 12–15 minutes until golden brown. Allow to cool for just 5 minutes on the baking tray, then turn out onto a wire rack while they are still warm but not hot, and leave to cool completely. Once cold, store in an airtight container.

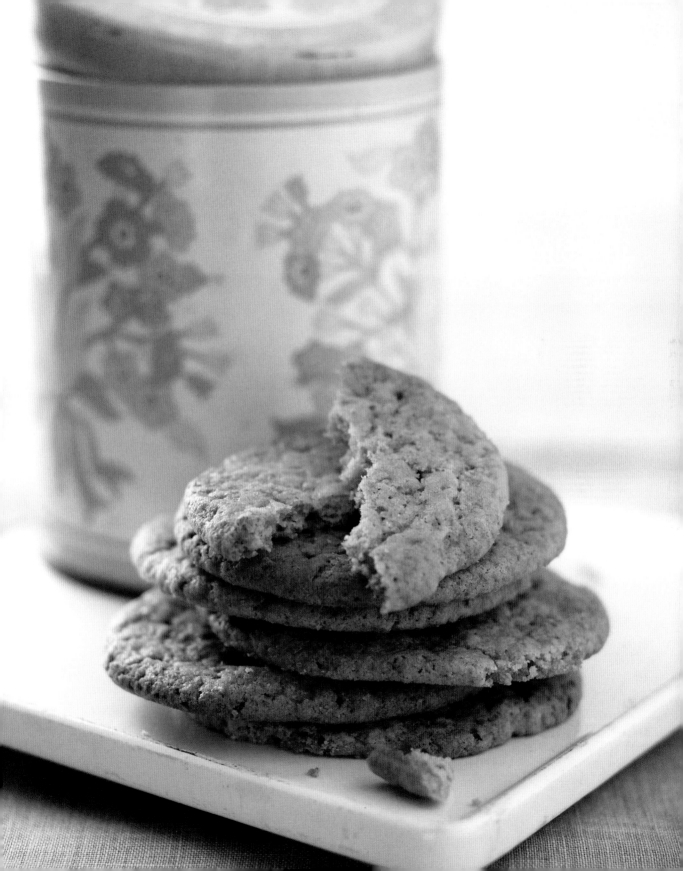

Gooey Chocolate Orange Cookies

Gorgeously gooey in the middle, these cookies are made using low-fat spread instead of butter and there is not a chemical enhancement in sight! They are perfect to make with that traditional Christmas stocking chocolate orange.

MAKES 18 COOKIES

250g (9oz) low-fat, heart-
  healthy spread
55g (2oz) caster sugar
85g (3oz) dark muscovado
  sugar
275g (10oz) self-raising
  flour
2 tbsp skimmed milk
55g (2oz) hazelnuts,
  chopped
175g (6oz) orange-
  flavoured chocolate,
  chopped

1 Preheat the oven to 180°C/350°F/Gas mark 4.

2 Line 2 large baking sheets with non-stick baking parchment.

3 In a large bowl, beat the low-fat spread and the sugars together using a wooden spoon until the mixture is light and fluffy. You might need to use the back of a fork to crush any lumps in the muscovado sugar.

4 Now, sift in the flour, add the milk and mix everything together with the wooden spoon.

5 Next, stir in the chopped nuts and chocolate and combine well.

6 Divide the mixture into 16 portions and shape each into a rough ball using slightly damp hands to prevent sticking. Place the balls onto the prepared baking sheets, making sure they are spaced well apart and flatten each ball with the back of a fork.

7 Bake for 15–20 minutes until golden around the edges but still pale and soft in the middle. Allow to cool for just 5 minutes on the baking trays before transferring to a wire rack to cool completely. These will keep well in an airtight container for up to 5 days.

Chocolate Pistachio Biscuits

Twice baked – twice as nice! These biscuits are like Italian biscotti and are absolutely delicious. Serve with a lovely cup of coffee or hot chocolate or on the side of a yogurt and fruit dessert – perfect.

MAKES 24

175g (6oz) good-quality plain dark chocolate, broken into pieces
2 tbsp low-fat, heart-healthy spread
300g (10½oz) self-raising flour, plus extra for dusting
1½ tsp baking powder
85g (3oz) caster sugar
55g (2oz) dry polenta
finely grated rind of 1 lemon
1 egg, lightly beaten
85g (3oz) shelled, unsalted pistachio nuts, roughly chopped
2 tbsp icing sugar, for dusting

1 Preheat the oven to 160°C/315°F/Gas mark 2–3.

2 Line a baking tray with greaseproof paper or a non-stick silicone sheet.

3 To melt the chocolate you can either put the broken pieces of chocolate and low-fat spread into a heatproof bowl set over a saucepan of simmering water and stir continuously until melted and smooth, or place the chocolate and low-fat spread in a microwavable bowl and melt in the microwave for 20 seconds at a time, stirring and checking in between each 20 second blast. You want to be careful that the chocolate doesn't burn.

4 Now, in another large bowl, sift the flour and baking powder together, then mix in the caster sugar, dry polenta, grated lemon rind, beaten egg and chopped pistachios. Add the melted chocolate and stir together to form a soft dough.

5 Lightly dust your hands with flour, then divide the dough in half and shape each piece into a 28cm (11in) long sausage.

recipe continues...

TIP
These biscuits will keep for
about a week in an airtight
container.

6   Transfer the 2 biscuit tubes onto the prepared baking tray and flatten slightly with the palm of your hand to about 2cm (¾in) thick.

7   Bake for 20 minutes until firm to the touch. Leave the oven on. Allow to cool on the baking tray for 8–10 minutes. When cooled but not cold, transfer to a chopping board and carefully slice diagonally into thin biscuits.

8   Now, put these biscuits back onto the baking tray, return to the oven and cook for a further 10 minutes until crisp to the touch.

9   This time, cool on a wire rack until completely cold, then dust with icing sugar and serve.

Crunchy Nut Fingers

With no added butter, these healthy, crunchy biscuits will keep everyone happy and filled up when lunch is still a way away. I love using dried apricots in desserts, as they add a wonderful sweetness and a delicious gooey-ness that is irresistible.

MAKES 16

2 eggs
200g (7oz) golden
  caster sugar
seeds from 1 vanilla pod
½ tsp ground cinnamon
½ tsp ground allspice
60g (2¼oz) ready-to-eat
  dried apricots, finely
  chopped
175g (6oz) ground almonds
125g (4½oz) hazelnuts,
  very finely chopped
  in a food processor
½ tsp baking powder
50g (1¾oz) flaked almonds

TIP
These biscuits can
be stored in an airtight
container for up to a week.

1 Preheat the oven to 140°C/275°F/Gas mark 1.

2 Line 2 baking trays with non-stick baking parchment or a cooking sheet.

3 Using a free-standing electric mixer, whisk the eggs, sugar and vanilla seeds until the mixture is pale and doubled in volume. This will take about 5 minutes of whisking.

4 Using a large, metal spoon, fold in the spices, chopped apricots, ground almonds, chopped hazelnuts and baking powder.

5 Spoon the mixture into a large piping bag fitted with a 1cm (½in) plain nozzle and pipe the mixture into 5cm (2in) long fingers onto the prepared baking trays, making sure you leave a little space for the biscuits to spread.

6 Gently press the flaked almonds on the top of each biscuit and bake for about 30 minutes until lightly golden.

7 Remove from the oven and transfer to a wire rack to cool.

Chocolate-dipped Meringue Fingers

These brilliant little sweet treats will satisfy a sweet tooth without overloading on fat. You can store them in an airtight container for 4 or 5 days... if they last that long!

MAKES 15

1 egg white
4 tbsp caster sugar
1½ tbsp cocoa powder, sifted
140g (5oz) good-quality plain dark chocolate, broken into pieces

TIP
Try serving these chocolate-dipped fingers with a fruit salad for an added treat.

1   Preheat the oven to 120°C/250°F/Gas mark ½.

2   Line a baking tray with greaseproof paper or a non-stick silicone sheet.

3   In a small clean bowl, whisk the egg white until it forms soft peaks.

4   Next, whisk half the sugar and continue whisking until stiff and glossy.

5   Using a metal spoon or spatula, fold in the remaining sugar and the sifted cocoa, then spoon the mixture into a piping bag fitted with a 1cm (½in) round nozzle and pipe fingers about 7.5 cm (3in) long onto the prepared baking sheet, spacing them about 2.5cm (1in) apart.

6   Bake for 1 hour until completely dry throughout. Allow to cool on a wire rack.

7   To coat the fingers in chocolate, put the chopped chocolate in a heatproof bowl set over a saucepan of simmering water and stir continuously until the chocolate has melted and is smooth. Remove from the heat and allow to cool slightly.

8   Once the meringues are completely cool, dip each end of the finger in the chocolate and place on baking parchment to set.

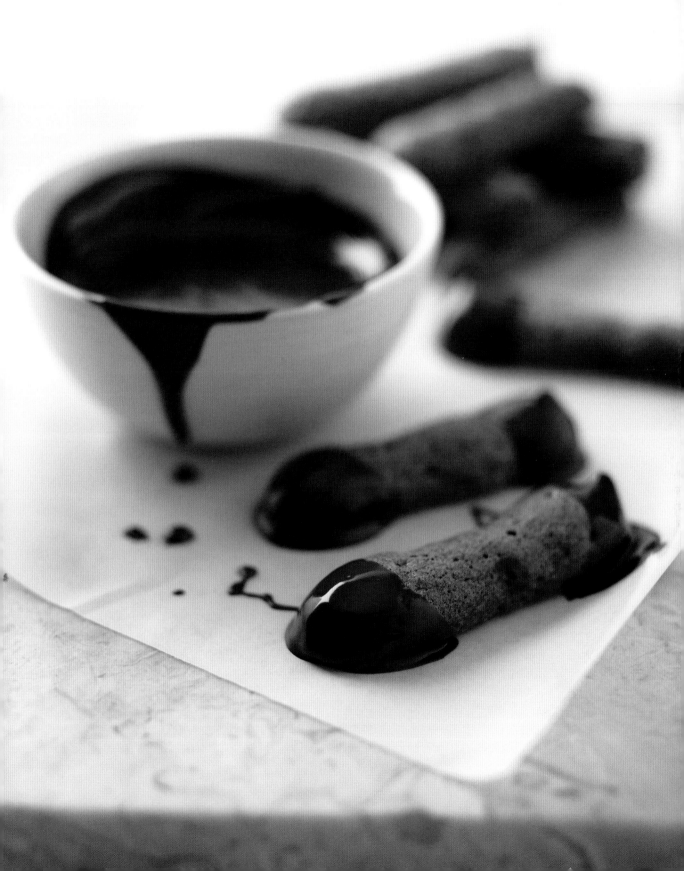

Energy Bites

These are wonderful little energy cookies – perfect for kids' lunch boxes or your mid-morning snack. Barley flakes are a bit crispier than oat flakes and are available from most health food shops, but if you can't get hold of them, oat flakes will do just fine.

MAKES 16 COOKIES

50g (1¾oz) hazelnuts
  or pecan nuts,
  finely chopped
50g (1¾oz) sunflower
  seeds, finely chopped
50g (1¾oz) ready-to-eat
  dried apricots, finely
  chopped
50g (1¾oz) raisins,
  finely chopped
1 tbsp light muscovado
  sugar
50g (1¾oz) barley flakes
50g (1¾oz) wholemeal
  self-raising flour
½ tsp baking powder
2 tbsp sunflower oil
4 tbsp apple juice

TIP
These cookies will keep
for 4 or 5 days in an
airtight container –
if they last that long!

1 Preheat the oven to 190°C/375°F/Gas mark 5.

2 Line a large baking sheet with baking parchment.

3 Mix the chopped nuts, sunflower seeds, apricots and raisins together in a bowl.

4 Next, add the sugar, barley flakes, flour and baking powder and stir until everything is thoroughly combined. There is no need to sift the flour – this is a rough-and-ready recipe!

5 Now, add the sunflower oil and apple juice and mix together. Don't expect this to be a smooth mixture – it will be a bit dry and clumpy.

6 Spoon out a heaped teaspoon of the mixture at a time, and with damp hands, roll into a ball and flatten slightly with the palm of your hand. Each cookie should measure roughly about 5cm (2in) in diameter.

7 Place each cookie on the prepared baking sheet, making sure they are spaced well apart because they will spread during cooking, and bake for 10–15 minutes until slightly risen and golden brown.

8 Remove from the oven and transfer to a wire rack to cool.

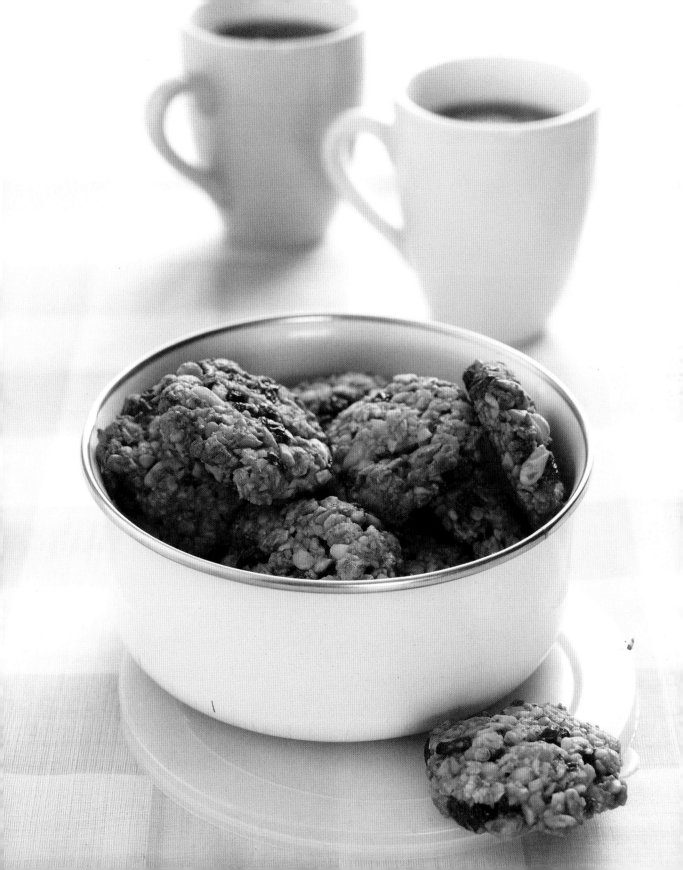

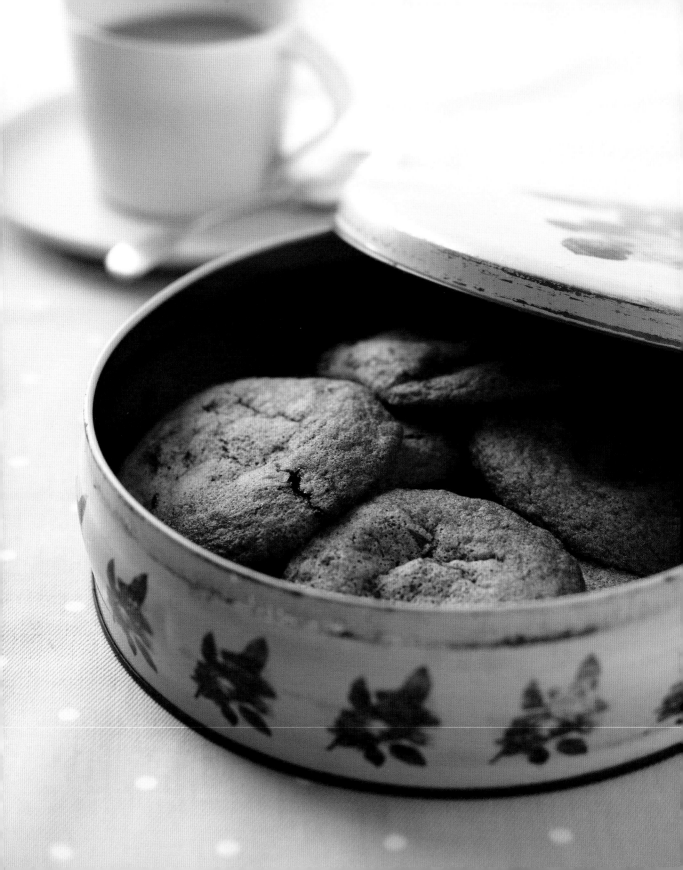

Gluten-free Cookies

The gluten-free ingredients for these cookies can be bought at most large supermarkets, but if you are struggling to find them, you could look online. You have an option here of using either low-fat, heart-healthy spread or butter – the choice is yours.

MAKES 8 COOKIES

100g (3½oz) golden
   caster sugar
100g (3½oz) soft
   brown sugar
50g (1¾oz) low-fat,
   heart-healthy spread
   or butter
2 eggs, beaten
1 tsp vanilla extract
3 tsp gluten-free
   bicarbonate of soda
2 tsp ground cinnamon
1 tsp ground ginger
200g (7oz) white rice flour
75g (2½oz) gluten-free
   chocolate chips

TIP
Once completely cooled,
store in an airtight
container for 2–3 days.

1   Preheat the oven to 180°C/350°F/Gas mark 4.

2   Line a large baking sheet with non-stick
    baking parchment.

3   Using a free-standing electric mixer, combine both the
    sugars and the spread or butter until starting to go pale.

4   Now, add the eggs and vanilla extract to the mixture
    and whizz up until very well blended.

5   Next, sift the bicarbonate of soda, cinnamon,
    ginger, and white rice flour into another bowl and
    mix together with a wooden spoon until they are
    combined. Add the sugar mixture and mix well.

6   Finally add the chocolate chips and stir, making sure
    the chocolate chips are evenly distributed through
    the mixture.

7   Now, using a medium-sized spoon, place rounded
    spoonfuls of the mixture onto the prepared baking
    sheet and bake in the oven for 12–15 minutes. Remove
    from the oven and transfer straight onto a wire rack
    to cool.

Italian Diamonds

We all love these slightly crunchy, slightly chews diamonds and they remind me of the Turkish biscuits we had at our wedding. So, make them with love! If you can't find the edible rice paper, use non-stick baking parchment instead. These cookies are best eaten on the day they are made.

MAKES 12

125g (4½oz) blanched
  almonds
grated zest from
  1 unwaxed lemon
15g (½oz) plain flour
1 tsp baking powder
60g (2¼oz) caster sugar
1 large egg white
100g (3½oz) icing sugar,
  plus extra for dusting
50g (1¾oz) cornflour
edible rice paper for lining
  the baking tray

To serve
strawberries and
  raspberries
low-fat crème fraîche

1 Preheat the oven to 140°C/275°F/Gas mark 1.

2 Put the almonds, lemon zest, plain flour and baking powder into a food processor and blitz to form a paste.

3 Now, put the caster sugar and 4 teaspoons of water in a small saucepan and bring to the boil. Reduce the heat and simmer for 2–3 minutes or until reduced to a thick syrup. Remove the saucepan from the heat and add the almond paste. Mix together thoroughly using a wooden spoon. Leave this mixture to cool for 1 hour.

4 Using a free-standing electric mixer, whisk the egg white and 1 teaspoon of the icing sugar until stiff and glossy.

5 Add the almond paste mixture to the whisked egg white and, using a large metal spoon, gently fold together until combined.

6 Have your prepared baking sheet lined with rice paper on hand. Sift the remaining icing sugar and the cornflour onto a clean work surface, turn out the mixture and roll into a log shape about 6cm (2½in) thick, then flatten until it is 4cm (1½in) thick.

7 Cut into 1cm (½in) slices, place on the prepared baking sheet and use a knife to cut into a diamond shape. Bake for about 30 minutes or until risen but still soft in the middle. Allow to cool on the baking sheet for 3–4 minutes, then transfer to a wire rack to cool.

8 Serve with a dusting of icing sugar and a helping of fresh strawberries and raspberries with some low-fat crème fraîche on the side.

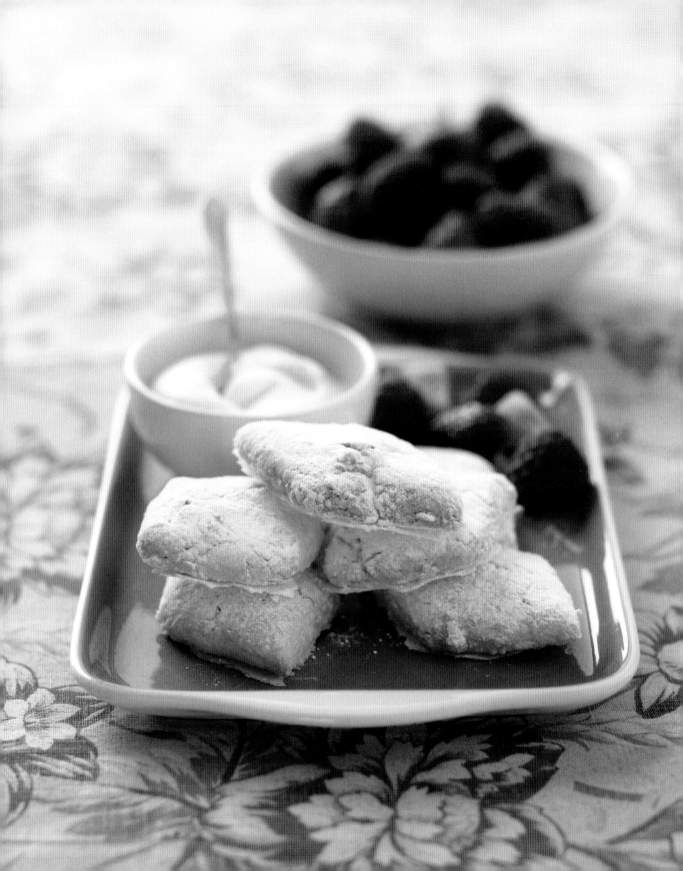

Squishy Flapjacks

The butter is replaced by the naturally sweet apricot purée in these delicious, glistening, squishy delights. My children enjoy these in their lunch boxes as an after-school snack and, would you believe it, in a bowl with custard! Try it – you might like it.

MAKES 8

250g (9oz) ready-to-eat
  dried apricots,
  cut into quarters
400ml (14fl oz) orange
  juice or apple juice
grated zest of ½ lemon
50g (1¾oz) crystallised
  ginger, finely chopped
200g (7oz) rolled oats
3 tbsp dark muscovado
  sugar
25g (1oz) raisins (optional)
25g (1oz) sunflower seeds

TIP
You can store your
flapjacks for 3–4 days
in an airtight container.

1 Preheat the oven to 180°C/350°F/Gas mark 4.

2 Line the base of a 22 cm (8½in) round loose-bottom cake tin with non-stick baking parchment.

3 Place the apricots, orange juice and lemon zest in a large saucepan over a high heat and bring to the boil. Reduce the heat and simmer, uncovered and stirring occasionally, for 25–30 minutes until the liquid is absorbed.

4 In a food processor or in the saucepan with a hand-held blender, purée the apricot mixture until smooth.

5 Now, stir the chopped ginger, oats, sugar, raisins (if using) and sunflower seeds into the apricot purée and mix well. Tip the mixture into the tin, spread out evenly and press down gently with the back of a metal spoon.

6 Bake for 30–35 minutes until firm and golden brown. Allow to cool slightly for 5–10 minutes before removing the base from the cake tin and cutting into wedges. Leave the flapjack to cool completely before lifting the wedges off the base.

Wholemeal Bran Cookies

Another healthy treat that will fill you up. These cookies are so much better for you than shop-bought biscuits, as all the ingredients are natural. These cookies are lovely plain but you may also want to try them with an addition of 2 tablespoons of dried fruit, currants or sultanas – add these at the kneading stage.

MAKES 36

300g (10½oz) wholemeal
   plain flour, plus extra
   for dusting
2 tbsp wheatgerm
¼ tsp bicarbonate of soda
50g (1¾oz) caster sugar
125g (4½oz) low-fat, heart-
   healthy spread, chilled
1 egg
1 tsp vanilla extract

TIP
These biscuits can
be stored in an airtight
container for a couple
of days.

1   Preheat the oven to 170°C/325°F/Gas mark 3.

2   Place the flour, wheatgerm, bicarbonate of soda and sugar in a large bowl and mix together.

3   Add the chilled low-fat spread and, using a knife, cut into the dry ingredients. Rub the spread into the flour mixture with your fingertips until the mixture resembles breadcrumbs.

4   In a cup, mix the egg with the vanilla extract with a fork, then add this to the breadcrumb mixture.

5   Use slightly damp hands to work the ingredients together to form a ball of dough. If it is still a little dry, add a small amount of cold water (if you are adding fruit – add it at this point).

6   Roll the dough out onto a lightly floured surface until it is about 1.5cm (⅝in) thick. Use a 7cm (2¾in) cookie cutter to cut out the biscuits and place them on a non-stick baking sheet, leaving a space between each one to allow for spreading during cooking. If your baking sheet isn't big enough, bake in batches for 20–25 minutes or until the biscuits are dry but not browned.

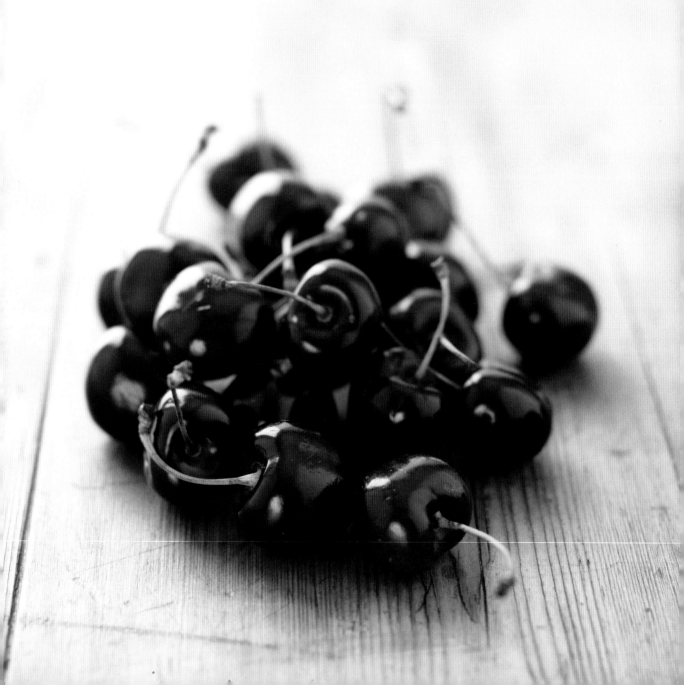

COOL PUDS

Tropical Fruit Pavlova

I sometimes use liquid egg whites, bought in a carton, for this recipe so I don't end up wasting all the yolks. This pavlova is fat-free and loaded with fruit – happy days!

SERVES 8

200ml (7fl oz) free-range liquid egg white (available in most supermarkets) or 5 egg whites
250g (9oz) caster sugar
300ml (10fl oz) low-fat crème fraîche or fat-free Greek yogurt
1 ripe mango, peeled and sliced
½ papaya, peeled, deseeded and sliced
½ sweet pineapple, peeled and cubed
1 kiwi fruit, peeled and thinly sliced
100g (3½oz) strawberries, halved

1 Preheat the oven to 140°C/275°F/Gas mark 1.

2 Draw a 25cm (10in) circle on a sheet of baking parchment and place on a baking sheet. Make sure to turn the paper over before lining the baking sheet so that you don't get pencil lead on your pudding!

3 In a large, clean bowl, whisk the liquid egg whites with an electric whisk until it forms soft peaks. Keep whisking while gradually adding the caster sugar until it is very stiff and glossy and shiny.

4 I like to use a piping bag to make the pavlova, but it works just as well using a palette knife to spread the egg mixture on top of the drawn circle in an even layer but building up slightly around the edges.

5 Bake for 2–3 hours, then switch the oven off and leave inside the oven to completely dry out for up to another hour. You want the meringue to remain pale but be completely dried on the outside 'crust'. remove from the oven and allow to cool completely.

6 Just before serving, spread the low-fat crème fraîche or fat-free Greek yogurt on top of the meringue and scatter with all the delicious chopped fruit. Feel free to add any extra fruit you have available and pile it up high!

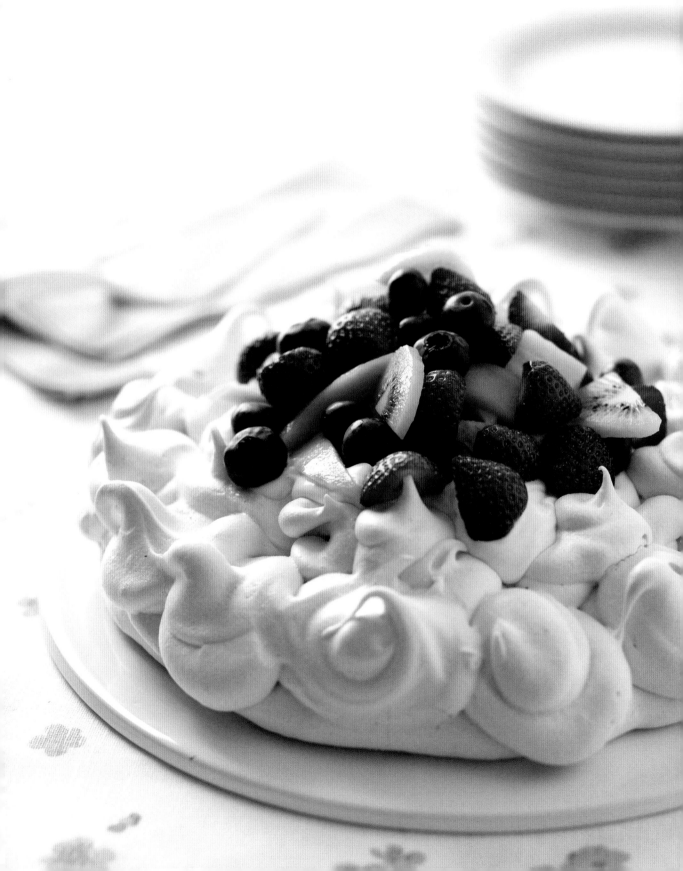

Banana & Coconut Cream Tart

This is a strange one for me because I don't like bananas (I wish I did) or coconut, but I love this tart. It's a great one to make for guests because it looks really impressive and tastes even better than it looks!

MAKES A 23CM (9IN) TART

For the tart case
225g (8oz) whole pecan
    nuts
275g (10oz) ready-to-eat
    pitted dates
2 tsp maple syrup

For the cream filling
150g (5½oz) raw cashew
    nuts, soaked overnight
    and thoroughly drained
2 tbsp plus 2 tsp maple
    syrup, and more to taste
1 vanilla pod, split in half
    lengthways
70g (3oz) desiccated
    coconut
4 ripe but firm bananas

1 To make the tart case, using a food processor or blender, coarsely chop the pecans. Add the dates and pulse until thoroughly combined, about 15–20 seconds.

2 Now, add the maple syrup and pulse again, until just combined and the mixture easily sticks together.

3 Using the back of a metal spoon and your damp hand, press the nut mixture firmly and evenly into a 23cm (9in) ceramic pie dish and pop the tart case into the refrigerator to set.

4 To make the filling, grind the cashew nuts to a coarse paste in a food processor or blender. Add 125ml (4fl oz) water, the maple syrup and the vanilla pod scrapings and blend until smooth, scraping the sides as needed. The mixture should be the consistency of thick pancake batter.

5 Reserve 2 tablespoons of the desiccated coconut and add the remainder to the blender, and blitz to combine. Pour the filling mixture into the chilled prepared tart case, spreading it evenly.

6 Next, peel and thinly slice the bananas on the bias and arrange in slightly overlapping rows, beginning at the edge of the tart. Sprinkle with the reserved desiccated coconut and serve immediately.

Caramelised Apples

This recipe makes a wonderful accompaniment to pancakes or porridge for breakfast or with low-fat yogurt or ice cream for dessert. I have kept the butter in this recipe, as it's such a small amount and the flavour is delicious.

SERVES 8

2 tsp butter
4 large apples (preferably Granny Smith), peeled, cored and cut into ½cm (1in) thick slices
2 tsp cornflour
75g (2½oz) soft dark brown sugar
½ tsp ground cinnamon

1 In a large, non-stick frying pan, melt the butter over a medium heat and add the sliced apples. Cook for 6–7 minutes, stirring and turning constantly, until the apples are almost tender.

2 In a cup, dissolve the cornflour in 125ml (4fl oz) cold water and add to the pan along with the brown sugar and cinnamon. Boil for 2 minutes, stirring occasionally, then remove from heat and serve warm.

Breakfast in a Glass

This is perfect to serve if you have overnight guests for breakfast, or we often have this as an after-school or after-work snack to keep us going until teatime, as it is so simple to make.

SERVES 2 LARGE GLASSES
OR 4 SMALL GLASSES

2 bananas
300ml (10fl oz) fruity low-fat bio yogurt
150g (5½oz) blueberries
400ml (14fl oz) cranberry juice
2–3 tbsp wheatgerm
1 tbsp clear honey, or to taste
flaked almonds, to decorate

1 Put all the ingredients except the honey and almonds in a blender and blitz until smooth.

2 Sweeten to taste with extra honey if desired, then pour into glasses and scatter over the almonds to decorate. Serve immediately.

Balsamic Strawberries

This is the best way to serve summer strawberries, as the balsamic vinegar brings out the strawberries' beautiful colour and really enhances their flavour.

SERVES 6

450g (1lb) fresh
   strawberries, hulled
   and cut in half
2 tbsp balsamic vinegar
50g (1¾oz) caster sugar
freshly ground black
   pepper, for sprinkling

1   Place the strawberries in a bowl. Drizzle the vinegar over the strawberries and sprinkle with the sugar. Stir gently to combine.

2   Cover with clingfilm, and leave to stand at room temperature for at least 1 hour but not more than 4 hours.

3   Just before serving, sprinkle with a little black pepper.

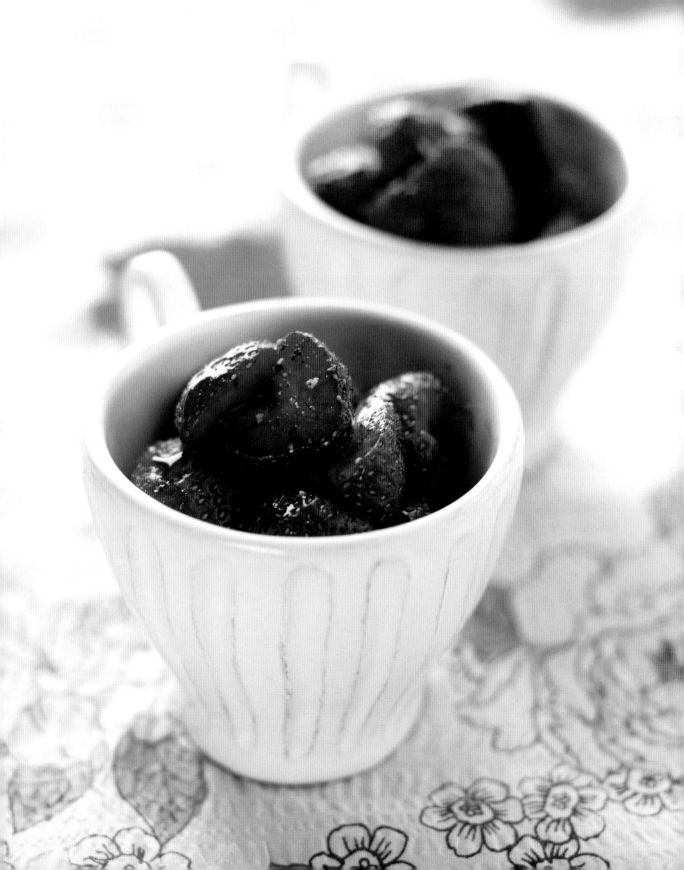

Blackcurrant Mousse

Made with egg whites, this mousse is incredibly light and fluffy and the perfect finale to a large meal. If you are feeding young children, pregnant women or the frail, omit the egg whites – it still makes a delicious dessert.

SERVES 4

1 x 12g (½oz) packet
  blackcurrant sugar-
  free jelly
juice of ½ lemon
290g (10oz) can
  blackcurrants in juice,
  drained and juice
  reserved
2 egg whites
150g (5½oz) low-fat
  plain yogurt

1   In a heatproof jug, sprinkle the jelly crystals into 200ml (7fl oz) boiling water, stirring to dissolve.

2   Add the lemon juice and the juice from the can of blackcurrants and, if necessary, add enough cold water to make the jelly up to 400ml (14fl oz). Pour the mixture into a large bowl and chill in the refrigerator for 30 minutes or until the jelly is starting to thicken.

3   In a separate clean bowl, whisk the egg whites until soft peaks form.

4   Now, stir the yogurt into the jelly, then fold in the egg whites using a large metal spoon. Spoon the jelly into 4 ramekins, cover with clingfilm and chill for 3 hours or until set.

5   To serve, spoon whole blackcurrants onto the top of each mousse.

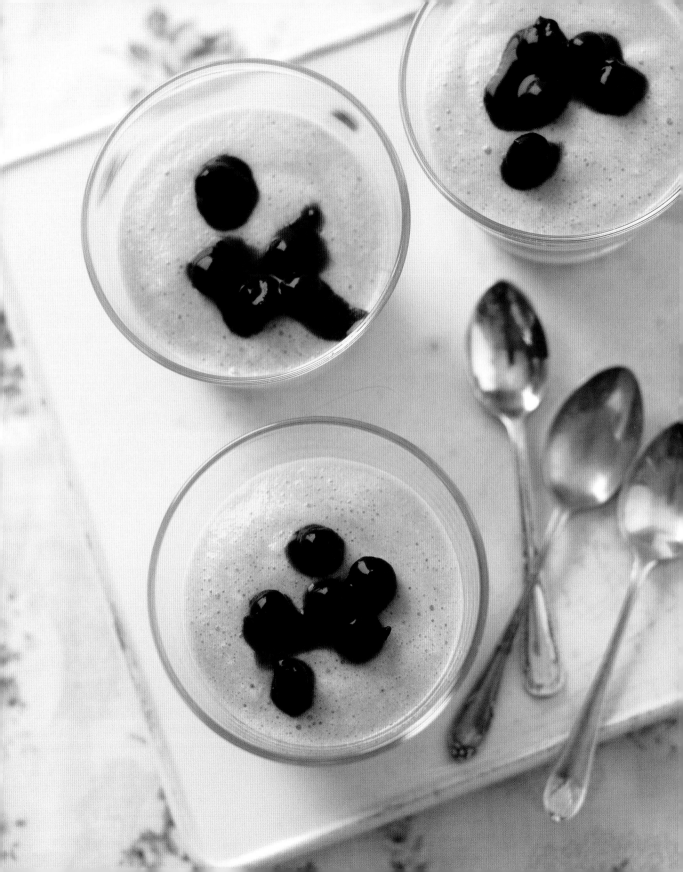

Brandy Snap & Berry Tower

OK, with this dish you can go to town. Have a competition and see who can build the highest tower – it looks amazing but is impossible to eat elegantly. Who cares!

SERVES 4

500g (1lb 2oz) mixed
   summer fruit, such
   as strawberries,
   blackberries, raspberries
   and blueberries
1 tbsp caster sugar

For the brandy snap rounds
50g (1¾oz) low-fat, heart-
   healthy spread
50g (1¾oz) golden syrup
50g (1¾oz) caster sugar
100g (3½oz) plain flour,
   plus extra for dusting
½ tsp ground ginger

For the vanilla cream
500ml (17fl oz) low-fat
   crème fraîche
1 tsp vanilla extract
1 tbsp icing sugar, sifted,
   plus extra for dusting

1   Preheat the oven to 190°C/375°F/Gas mark 5.

2   Draw a 20cm (8in) circle on 4 separate sheets of non-stick baking parchment and place each parchment sheet onto a flat baking sheet.

3   Put the fruit in a bowl, sprinkle with the 1 tablespoon of caster sugar, cover and set aside at room temperature.

4   To make the brandy snaps, gently melt the low-fat spread, golden syrup and caster sugar over a low heat in a large saucepan.

5   Remove from the heat and add the flour and ginger. Stir briefly with a wooden spoon to bring the mixture together to form a soft ball of dough.

6   Transfer the dough onto a very lightly floured surface and, using damp hands, divide the dough into 4 portions, then shape each piece into a ball.

7   While the dough is still warm, put a ball in the centre of each baking parchment template (make sure you have turned the paper over so that the pencil lead doesn't get on your snaps) and push out the dough with the heel of your hand. Cover with cling film and roll out with a rolling pin until you have a very thin round just covering the outline of the circle. Neaten the edge with a knife.

recipe continues...

8 Now, remove the clingfilm and bake 2 at a time for 4–6 minutes until golden brown (keep an eye on them, as they turn very quickly).

9 Slide the baking parchment off the baking sheets and cool the snaps on wire racks.

10 When cold and crisp, peel off the baking parchment.

11 To make the filling, in a bowl, whisk the crème fraîche, vanilla extract and sifted icing sugar together with a hand whisk.

12 Layer the brandy snap rounds with cream and fruit to form a stack. Top with a little fruit and sprinkle with icing sugar to serve.

Lemon Cream Pudding with Blackberries

This is a delicious alternative to a calorie-laden lemon torte. It is a perfect blend of creaminess and sweetness, and the lemon juice adds a perfect burst of tartness. This dessert can be made in advance and will last in the refrigerator for up to three days.

SERVES 4

175g (6oz) clear honey
1 x 350g (12oz) packet
  tofu, firm or extra-firm,
  drained
grated zest of 1 lemon
60ml (2fl oz) fresh lemon
  juice
145g (5oz) fresh
  blackberries
icing sugar, sifted,
  for sprinkling

1 Using a blender or food processor, blend the honey, tofu, grated lemon zest (keeping 1 teaspoon of grated zest behind) and lemon juice together until smooth. Scrape down the sides with a spatula to make sure that you don't miss any bits.

2 Divide the lemon cream evenly among 4 bowls or serving glasses.

3 Top each dessert with the blackberries, the remaining reserved grated lemon zest and a sprinkling of sifted icing sugar. Serve immediately or refrigerate until needed.

Low-fat Baked Lemon Cheesecake

Although still containing some fat, this is a lower-fat version of cheesecake, which tastes every bit as good. It is incredibly light and fluffy and divine, so, watch the portion sizes – this cheesecake should serve at least 16 portions!

SERVES 16

55g (2oz) low-fat digestive
  biscuits, crushed.
55g (2oz) low-fat, heart-
  healthy spread
55g (2oz) ground almonds
450g (1lb) low-fat cream
  cheese
140g (5oz) caster sugar
4 eggs
grated zest of 1 lemon
  or orange
1 tbsp lemon or orange
  juice
75ml (3 floz) crème fraîche
icing sugar, sifted,
  for dusting

1   Preheat the oven to 140°C/275°F/Gas mark 1.

2   Place the biscuits in a strong plastic bag and bash with a rolling pin to crush. Set aside.

3   Melt the low-fat spread in a saucepan over a low heat, then stir in the crushed biscuits and ground almonds. Press the mixture firmly into a 20cm (8in) loose-bottomed, round cake tin using a metal spoon and pop into the freezer while you prepare the rest of the cheesecake.

4   Using a free-standing electric mixer or food processor, blend the low-fat cream cheese, sugar, eggs, grated zest, lemon or orange juice and the crème fraiche together. It will look a bit sloppy, but don't worry.

5   Remove the biscuit base from the freezer and pour the cheese mixture on top. Slide the cake tin carefully into the oven and cook for 45 minutes–1 hour. Check regularly throughout cooking; the centre will be slightly wobbly but set and not runny when done.

6   Allow to cool in the tin – it will firm more as it cools – then chill for at least an hour before dusting with a little sifted icing sugar and serving.

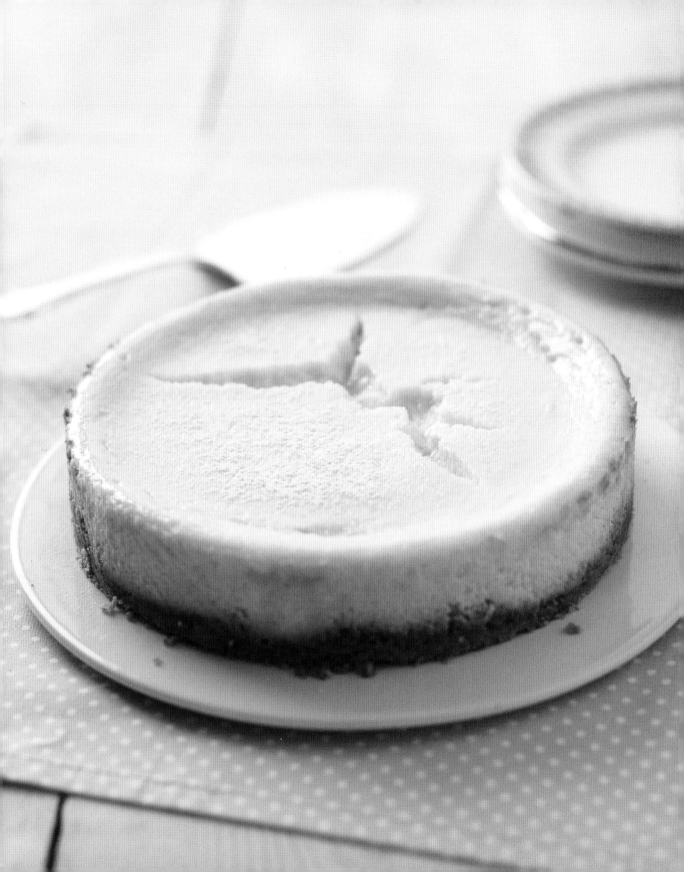

Mint Tea & Raspberry Jellies

Simple and easy to make but very pretty and tasty, these individual jellies brighten up a tea table and are refreshingly different.

SERVES 4

10 mint leaves, torn, plus extra 4 leaves to decorate
1 x 12g (½oz) packet raspberry sugar-free jelly
125g (4½oz) raspberries, thawed if frozen

1   Place the 10 torn mint leaves in a heatproof jug, pour over 300ml (10fl oz) boiling water and leave to infuse for 5 minutes

2   Add the jelly crystals to the jug and stir to dissolve.

3   Reserve 8 raspberries for the decoration and roughly crush the rest with the back of a fork. Stir the crushed raspberries into the jelly and top up with enough cold water to make 600ml (1 pint).

4   Divide the jelly among 4 glasses, then cool, uncovered, in the refrigerator for 2 hours or until set.

5   When ready to serve, decorate each dessert with 2 whole raspberries and a mint leaf on top of each jelly.

Watermelon & Honeydew Jelly

This is a great way to serve up melon. Made into a jelly 'loaf', sliced and served with some low-fat crème fraîche or Greek yogurt – this is a super-healthy and delicious light pudding.

SERVES 6-8

1 cantaloupe melon
  (about 1.4kg/3lb),
  halved and deseeded
1 wedge watermelon
  (about 900g/2lb),
  deseeded
750ml (1¼pints) apple juice
  or apple cider
4 sheets gelatine
85g (3oz) clear honey

1. Scoop out the melons with a melon baller and put straight into a 23 x 12cm (9 x 5in) non-stick loaf tin and set aside.

2. In a medium saucepan, bring the apple juice or cider (if using), 225ml (8fl oz) water and gelatine to the boil. Reduce the heat and simmer until the gelatine is dissolved, about 5 minutes.

3. Remove from the heat and use a wooden spoon to stir in the honey until dissolved.

4. Allow to cool to room temperature in the pan for about 40 minutes, then pour the cooled liquid over the melon balls and leave to set in the refrigerator, uncovered for about 3 hours.

5. To serve, turn the jelly out onto a platter and slice into individual portions.

Pineapple, Raspberry & Amaretti Parfaits

These parfaits will take just two minutes to prepare, but they are delicious –
sometimes the most simple things taste the best!

12 Amaretti biscuits
2 x 225g (8oz) container
  fat-free peach yogurt
1 punnet of fresh
  raspberries,
  (approximately
  150g/5½oz)
100g fresh or canned
  pineapple chunks

1   Place 2 Amaretti biscuits, broken into pieces, into the
    base of each of 4 decorative serving glasses.

2   Now, layer the yogurt and fruit and include another
    layer of biscuits, this time keeping the biscuit whole.

3   Finish with a layer of fruit on top and keep in the
    refrigerator until ready to serve.

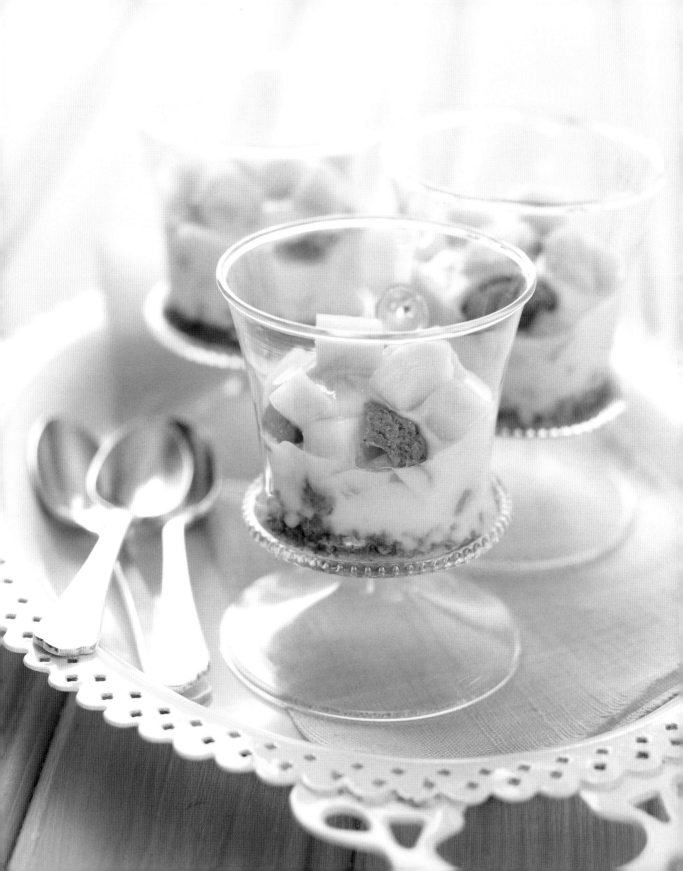

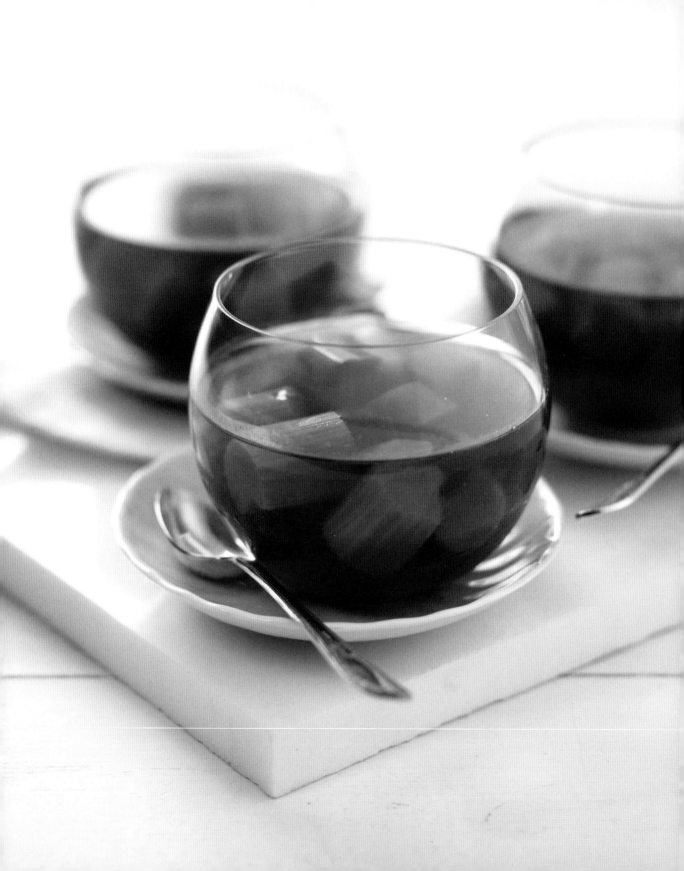

Pomegranate & Rhubarb Jelly

Here are some flavours you might not have put together in a jelly – but try this and you'll be hooked. The fresh ginger and rhubarb give a lovely tangy flavour and the pomegranate juice makes it heart healthy too.

SERVES 4

400g (14oz) fresh rhubarb, trimmed and cut into 2cm (¾in) chunks
40g (1½oz) caster sugar
20g (¾oz) fresh root ginger, peeled and grated
250ml (9fl oz) concentrated pomegranate juice
4 leaves gelatine

1 Place the rhubarb, sugar and grated ginger into a heavy-based lidded saucepan.

2 In a jug, mix the pomegranate juice with 750ml (1¼ pints) water, then add this mixture to the rhubarb, cover and cook over a medium heat for 7–8 minutes until the rhubarb is soft. Bring to the boil and boil for 5 minutes.

3 During this time, pop the gelatine leaves into a bowl of cold water for 5 minutes to soften.

4 After 5 minutes of bubbling, take the rhubarb mixture off the heat, remove the gelatine from the water, squeezing out any excess liquid, and add the gelatine to the rhubarb mixture. Stir thoroughly with a wooden spoon for 1 minute or until the gelatine has dissolved.

5 Allow to cool for about 20 minutes at room temperature, then pour the jelly mixture into 4 glasses or moulds. Put into the fridge, uncovered, and leave to set for 4–6 hours, then serve.

Simnel Tart

Marzipan is an acquired taste, and if you are a fan, this tart is rich in energy-giving almonds. The raisins provide the gorgeous sweetness, and the whole is surrounded in a light, crispy puff pastry.

SERVES 6

200g (7oz) mixed dried
  fruit
3 tbsp chopped mixed nuts
grated zest and juice of
  1 orange
1 x 375g (13oz) sheet
  ready-rolled 'light'
  puff pastry
3 tbsp low-sugar orange
  marmalade
200g (8oz) marzipan,
  grated
1 tbsp demerara sugar
low-fat crème fraîche,
  to serve

1 Preheat the oven to 200°C/400°F/Gas mark 6.

2 Line a baking sheet large enough to take the puff pastry sheet with greaseproof paper. Some of the shop-bought puff pastry now comes on its own greaseproof paper sheet, which is very helpful.

3 Mix the dried fruit, chopped mixed nuts, orange zest and juice together in a bowl and set aside. (My grandmother used to add a drop of brandy at this point – but I couldn't possibly comment on that!)

4 Unroll the puff pastry onto the prepared baking sheet and, using the edge of a knife, mark a frame all the way around, about 2cm (¾in) from the edge.

5 Brush the marmalade onto the inside section of the pastry. If it is difficult to brush, try melting for 10 seconds in a microwave first.

6 Now, drain the fruit and nuts through a sieve and pop into a bowl. Pour the juice into a small saucepan, as this is going to be reduced to make the glaze for around the edge of the tart.

7 Next, stir the grated marzipan into the fruit mixture and scatter this mixture on top of the jam and spread evenly. Leave the 2cm (¾in) border clear.

recipe continues...

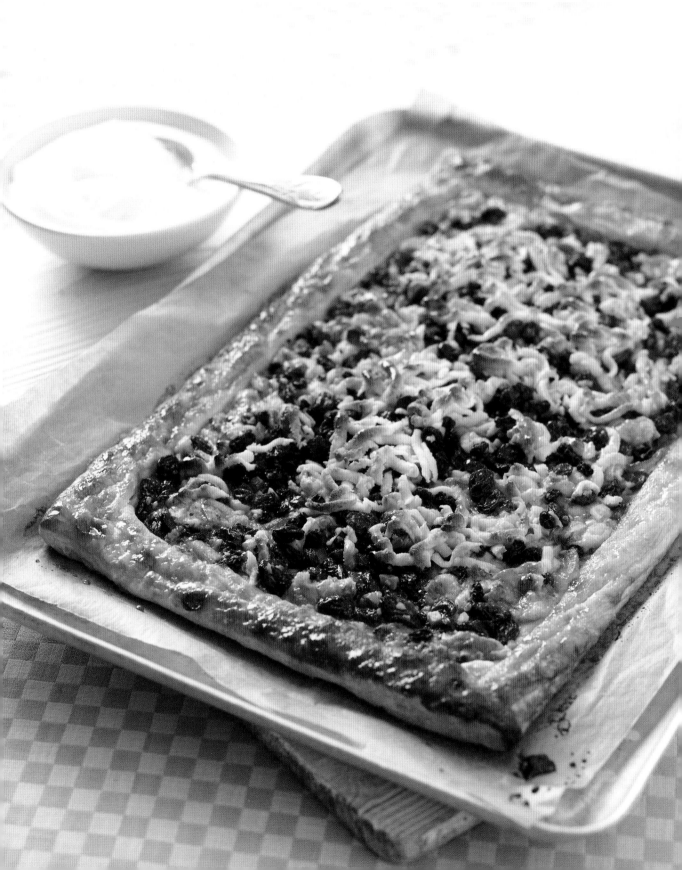

8 Finally, add the 1 tablespoon of demerara sugar to the orange juice and simmer over a low heat for 3–4 minutes until reduced and syrupy. Remove from the heat and brush around the border of the pastry to give a glistening, sweet glaze.

9 Bake for 20 minutes until the pastry around the edge is risen and golden. Cut into squares and serve with some low-fat crème fraîche.

Strawberry Palmiers

These are delightfully light French pastries that can be adapted to suit your taste. I've made them here using strawberries but you can use any in-season fruit that you fancy. I've substituted the usual high-calorie fresh cream for low-fat soft cheese mixed with a little icing sugar. Or you can substitute the soft cheese for 'squirty' low-fat cream.

MAKES 8

7 tbsp caster sugar
1 x 400g (14oz) packet
   frozen 'light' puff pastry,
   thawed
200g (7oz) low-fat
   soft cheese
1 tbsp lemon juice
4 tbsp icing sugar,
   plus extra for dusting
225g (8oz) strawberries,
   cut in half

1 Preheat the oven to 220°C/425°F/Gas mark 7.

2 Line several baking sheets with non-stick baking parchment.

3 Sprinkle a tablespoon of the caster sugar over the clean work surface and unroll the pastry on top, then sprinkle the surface of the pastry with 2 tablespoons of the caster sugar.

4 Now, roll the pastry out slightly until it is a rectangle of approximately 35 x 4cm (14 x 10in). Sprinkle with another 2 tablespoons of caster sugar, leaving a gap around the edge of about 2cm (¾in) and lightly press this sugar into the pastry using the palm of your hand.

recipe continues...

5 With a sharp knife, very lightly score a line widthways across the middle of the pastry. Then, starting at one short side, roll the pastry up, stopping at the score mark in the middle. Do the same on the opposite side.

6 Now, cut the pastry widthways into 1cm (½in) thick slices.

7 Place the pastries, cut side up, about 5cm (2in) apart on the prepared baking sheets and sprinkle lightly with another tablespoon of the caster sugar.

8 Bake for 12 minutes, then turn the pastries over and sprinkle with the remaining 1 tablespoon of caster sugar and bake for a further 5 minutes or until golden brown and glazed. Transfer to wire racks to cool completely.

9 For the cream, either use a low-fat 'squirty' cream or mix the low-fat cream cheese, lemon juice and icing sugar together in a bowl.

10 Sandwich the palmiers together with the cream and strawberries, then sprinkle with a little icing sugar and serve.

Chocolate Vanilla Mousse

This recipe was very kindly donated to me by the chocolate lady extraordinaire, Claire Burnet of Chococo. Thank you, Claire – we love it! Including a little good-quality milk chocolate just takes the edge off the intensity of pure dark chocolate for anyone wanting a little more sweetness. Even so, this recipe is still mostly dark chocolate and the flavour is suitably and beautifully delicious!

SERVES 4

200g (7oz) good-quality plain dark chocolate, ideally 70% cocoa solids or 150g (5½oz) plain dark chocolate and 50g (1¾oz) milk chocolate (minimum of 35% cocoa solids)
200ml (7fl oz) boiling water
1 tsp vanilla extract
cocoa powder, for dusting
crème fraîche fresh fruits or Chocolate Pistachio Biscuits (see page 87), to serve (optional)

NOTE
Any chocolate used must be made with pure cocoa butter and contain no added vegetable fats. Mousses made with just dark chocolate will set firmer than those made with the inclusion of milk chocolate as above.

1 Chop the chocolate into small chunks and place in a heatproof bowl set over a pan of barely simmering water, making sure the base of the bowl isn't touching the water and melt gently while stirring constantly.

2 Once the chocolate is melted, add 200ml (7fl oz) of just-boiled water (do not add water while it is still boiling, as it may scorch the chocolate), adding in thirds and stirring after each addition to form a smooth but quite runny mixture.

3 Stir in the vanilla extract. The mixture is very runny at this point but don't worry, it will thicken as it cools.

4 Pour this mixture into a lipped jug and then pour into small coffee cups or glasses. Using a lipped jug means you will be able to fill the cups easily without it dripping everywhere! These mousses are rich so you don't want big portions.

5 Put the mousses into the refrigerator to set for at least 1 hour but bring back to room temperature just before serving to soften to the right consistency.

6 To serve, dust with cocoa powder and serve as they are or with a dollop of crème fraîche, fresh berry fruits or my Chocolate Pistachio Biscuits.

FLAVOUR VARIATION
For a different flavour, you can make a tea infusion by adding a dessertspoon of aromatic loose leaf such as lapsang souchong, Moroccan mint or Earl Grey to the boiling water and strain onto the chocolate after infusing for 2 minutes.

Honey-walnut Turnovers

Turnovers remind me of my mum. When I was small, we used to go shopping together (which I loved) and we always used to buy a turnover from the baker's on the way home.

MAKES 30

200g (7oz) walnut halves
55g (2oz) caster sugar
grated zest of 1 lemon
½ tsp ground cinnamon
3 tbsp clear honey
2 tbsp reduced-sugar
 orange marmalade
20 sheets (23 x 35cm/
 9 x 14in) filo pastry
light cooking spray

For the glaze
1 egg, beaten
2 tbsp demerara sugar

1 Preheat the oven to 190°C/375°F/Gas mark 5.

2 Put the walnuts, caster sugar, lemon zest and cinnamon in a food processor and process until the walnuts are finely ground but not oily.

3 Next, add the honey and marmalade and blitz just for a few seconds to mix. Set aside.

4 Unroll the filo pastry onto a clean dry surface and cut it lengthways into 3 long strips, about 7.5 x 35cm (3 x 14in) each. Cover the pastry with a damp kitchen paper to prevent it from drying out as you work. (Remove the strips, as you need them, being sure to re-cover the remaining dough.)

5 Remove 2 strips of filo and stack one on top of the other, then spray the top strip with light cooking spray. Spread 2¼ teaspoons of the walnut filling over the bottom right-hand corner and fold the filled corner up and over to the left. Continue folding in this manner until you reach the end of the strip and form a triangle of dough. Repeat with the remaining filling and dough.

6 Spray a large baking sheet with cooking spray and arrange the pastries seam-side down on the sheet. To make the glaze, combine the beaten egg and demerara sugar in a small bowl and stir to mix.

7 Brush the glaze over the tops of the pastries. and bake for about 10–12 minutes or until golden brown. Let the pastries cool for at least 20 minutes before serving.

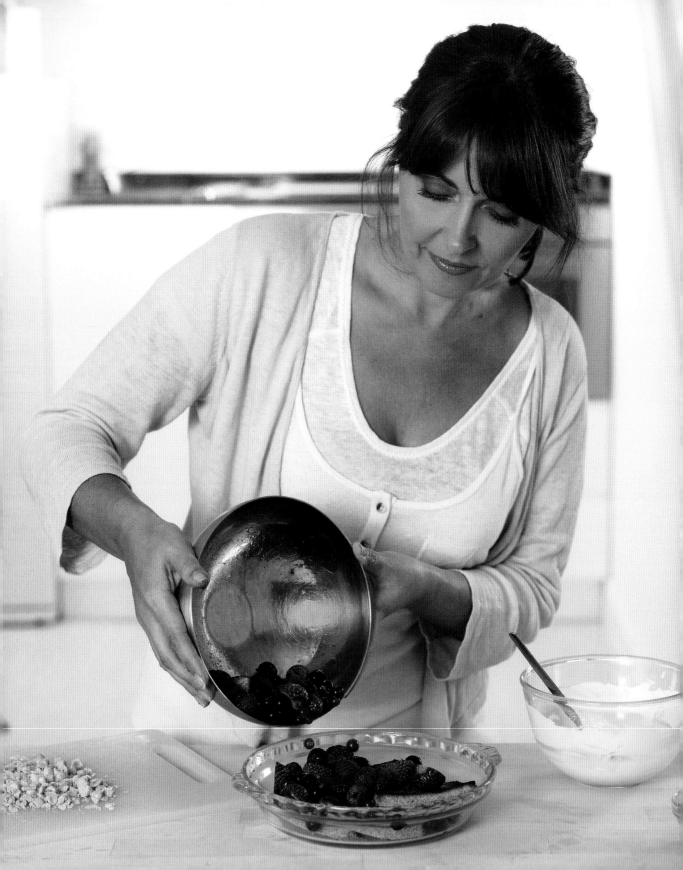

HOT DESSERTS

Guilt-free Sticky Toffee Puddings

This dessert is brilliant and you have to try it! It is great because it's butter-free, but do watch your portion sizes, as it contains lots of sugar and maple syrup. Serve with fat-free Greek yogurt and go for a big long walk after eating.

MAKES 4

low-fat spread,
  for greasing
175g (6oz) pitted
  dried dates
175ml (6fl oz) fresh
  orange juice
150ml (5fl oz) good-
  quality maple syrup
1 tbsp vanilla extract
2 eggs, separated
85g (3oz) self-raising
  flour, sifted
55g (2oz) pecan nuts,
  chopped
fat-free Greek yogurt,
  to serve

1   Preheat the oven to 180°C/350°F/Gas mark 4.

2   Grease 4 x 200ml (7fl oz) ramekins with low-fat spread.

3   Put the dates with 175ml (6fl oz) of orange juice in a pan and simmer for 5 minutes over a medium heat. Pour the date mixture into a food processor or liquidiser, add 6 tablespoons of the maple syrup and the vanilla extract and blend until smooth.

4   Transfer the mixture to a bowl and beat in the egg yolks and sifted flour with a wooden spoon until well combined.

5   In a separate, very clean bowl, whisk the eggs with an electric whisk until they form stiff peaks.

6   Now, use a large metal spoon or spatula to gently fold the stiff egg whites into the date mixture. Do not overmix. Stir in the chopped nuts.

7   Finally, put 1 tablespoon of maple syrup into each of the prepared ramekins and add the pudding mixture. Cover each of the ramekins tightly with kitchen foil, stand in a deep ovenproof dish and carefully pour enough hot water to come halfway up the sides of the ramekins.

8   Cook for 50 minutes–1 hour or until a skewer inserted into the centre of the pudding comes out clean.

9   To serve, tip the puddings upside down straight onto a serving plate and serve with a dollop of fat-free Greek yogurt.

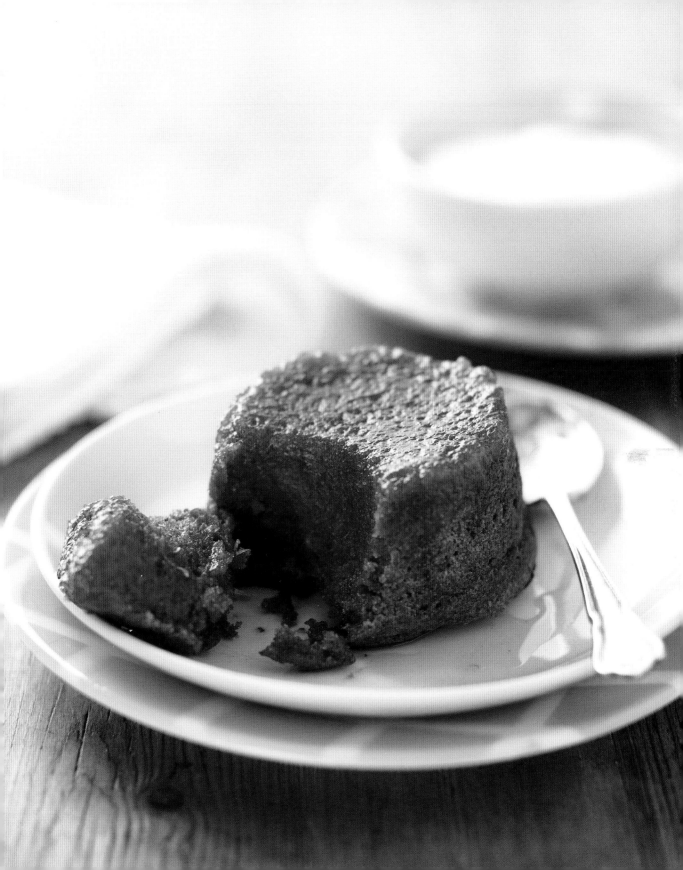

Tunisian Filo Pastries Stuffed with Dates

Try these delicious filled pastries for a dinner party dessert – they are simple to make but look very special and impressive! African countries have the most delectable desserts; they seem to go to so much trouble and the taste is always worth it.

MAKES 36

250g (9oz) ready-to-eat
  pitted dates
50g (1¾oz) blanched
  almonds, chopped
1 tsp ground cinnamon
Grated zest of ½ orange
2 egg yolks
400g (14oz) frozen filo
  pastry, thawed
75g (2½oz) low-fat, heart-
  healthy spread, melted
chopped pistachio nuts,
  for sprinkling

For the syrup
4 tbsp caster sugar
2 tbsp lemon juice
2 tbsp clear, runny honey

1 Preheat the oven to 180°C/350°F/Gas mark 4.

2 Line a baking tray with non-stick baking parchment.

3 Blend the dates in a food processor with 3 teaspoons water to make a soft paste. If the dates are very dry, put them in a saucepan with the water and warm over a low heat to soften, then blend in the food processor. If you buy ready-to-eat dates, they should be soft enough.

4 Now, add the almonds, cinnamon, grated orange zest and egg yolks and blend briefly.

5 Cut the filo into rectangles about 10cm (4in) wide by the width of the sheets. Put the rectangles of pastry in a pile and cover with a clean, damp tea towel so they don't dry out.

6 Working quickly, take one sheet at a time and brush it with the melted low-fat spread, then put 1 heaped teaspoonful of the filling at one end of the rectangle and spread into a line. Now, begin to roll the 'cigar', folding in the edges of the pastry over the filling about one-third of the way along. Finish rolling, without folding in the rest of the edges. Repeat this with each sheet of pastry.

recipe continues...

7   Arrange the pastries on the prepared baking tray and brush with the remaining low-fat spread. Bake in the oven for 30–40 minutes or until crisp and golden.

8   To make the syrup, put the sugar, lemon juice, honey and 6 tablespoons of water into a small saucepan and melt over a medium heat until the sugar and honey have dissolved.

9   As the pastries come out of the oven, pour over the syrup and sprinkle with chopped pistachios. Serve warm.

Cherry Clafoutis

Although considered a dessert, this dish was actually often served as a breakfast or brunch, so feel free to add to the menu at any time of the day. It is deliciously light and the cherries give it a healthy tick! If the cherries are too expensive, you can use small, sweet plums instead.

SERVES 8

1 tbsp butter or light
  cooking spray,
  for greasing or coating
450g (1lb) red cherries,
  pitted and halved
100g (3½oz) caster sugar
150g (5½oz) plain flour,
  sifted
2 eggs, beaten
300ml (10fl oz) skimmed
  milk
low-fat Greek yogurt,
  to serve

1 Preheat the oven to 190°C/375°F/Gas mark 5.

2 Grease a 1 litre (1¾ pint) shallow ovenproof dish with butter or spray with light cooking spray.

3 Place the prepared cherries, cut side down, in the base of the dish and sprinkle with 25g (1oz) of the caster sugar.

4 Now, place the sifted flour in a large bowl, make a well in the centre and add the beaten eggs and milk. Using a wooden spoon, gradually work the flour into the eggs and milk and beat to make a smooth batter. Stir in the remaining sugar and pour the batter over the cherries.

5 Bake in the oven for about 55 minutes or until well risen and firm to the touch. Serve warm with low-fat Greek yogurt.

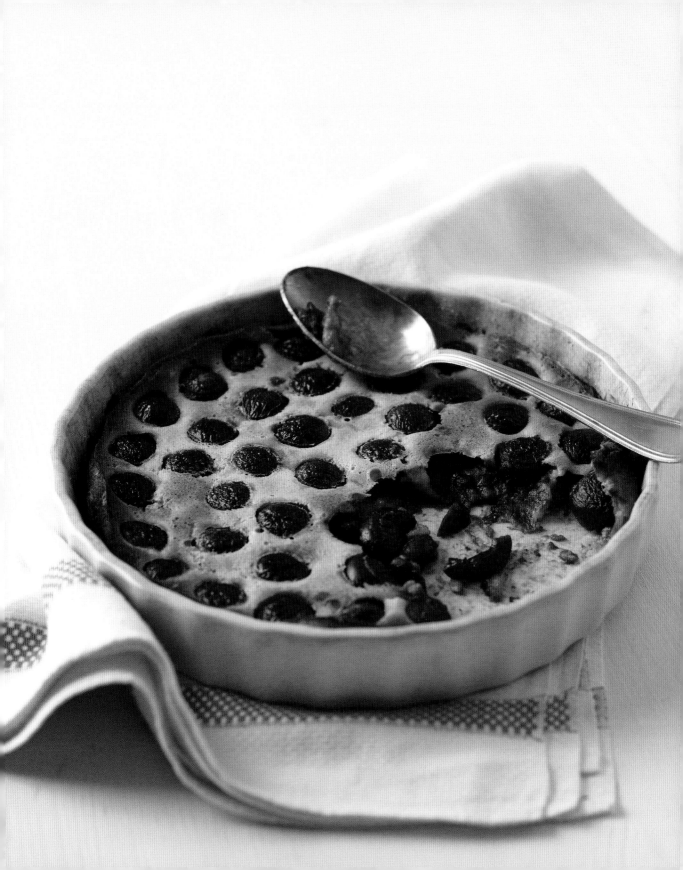

Apple & Prune Filo Pasty

Delicious flavours, light, low-fat pastry and quick and easy to make, these pasties remind me of the delicious little Turkish or Moroccan desserts – only healthier!

SERVES 6

3 tbsp English breakfast tea, hot – with no milk!
4 tbsp orange juice
225g (8oz) prunes, pitted (about 20)
6 eating apples, peeled and thickly sliced
25g (1oz) low-fat, heart-healthy spread
½ tsp ground cinnamon
6 tbsp caster sugar
grated zest of 1 lemon
6 sheets of filo pastry, thawed, covered with a clean, damp, tea towel
light cooking spray
4 tbsp finely chopped nuts (any kind but pecan nuts work well)
icing sugar, for dusting

1 Preheat the oven to 220°C/425°F/Gas mark 7.

2 Line a baking sheet with non-stick baking parchment.

3 Start by mixing the tea and orange juice together in a heatproof bowl. Add the prunes and allow to soak for about 2 hours, at room temperature.

4 In a large saucepan over a low heat, gently cook the prepared apples in the low-fat spread, the cinnamon, half the sugar and the lemon zest for 5 minutes.

5 Now, add the prunes and the marinade juices, then remove the pan from the heat and set aside.

6 Place 1 sheet of filo pastry on the prepared baking sheet. Leave the rest of the pastry covered in a clean damp tea towel. Spray the sheet of pastry that you are using lightly with the light cooking spray and place the next sheet on top at a slight angle, and spray lightly. Continue this process with all 6 sheets, arranging them so that the edges are all at angles and produce a pretty flower shape.

7 Sprinkle the chopped nuts into the centre of the pastry flower. Pile the apple and prune mixture, along with the juices, in the middle of the pastry and quickly gather the edges of the pastry in your fingers and

recipe continues...

bring it up and around the apple filling. You'll need to 'scrunch' the pastry together at the top to make a ruffle. Give one last spritz of cooking spray and dust with icing sugar.

8 Bake for 10 minutes, then lower the temperature to 180°C/350°F/Gas mark 4 and bake for a further 15–20 minutes until brown and crisp.

9 Sprinkle with a little more icing sugar and serve warm or cold.

Caribbean Bananas

Bananas are full of potassium, which is very good for the heart, and these baked bananas are so full of flavour, healthy eating has never tasted so good. Serve with some low-fat crème fraîche.

SERVES 8

low-fat, heart-healthy
  spread, for greasing
8 ripe bananas, peeled
  and cut in half lengthways
75g (3oz) soft brown sugar
125ml (4fl oz) fresh orange
  juice
½ tsp ground ginger
seeds from 4 cardamom
  pods, crushed
1 tsp ground allspice
low-fat crème fraîche,
  to serve

1 Preheat oven to 180°C/350°F/Gas mark 4.

2 Grease the base of a shallow baking dish with the low-fat spread.

3 Place the bananas cut-side down in the baking dish.

4 Mix the brown sugar, orange juice, ginger, crushed cardamom seeds and allspice together in a bowl and drizzle over the bananas.

5 Bake, uncovered, for 15 minutes until starting to brown and go syrupy around the edges. Serve warm with low-fat crème fraîche.

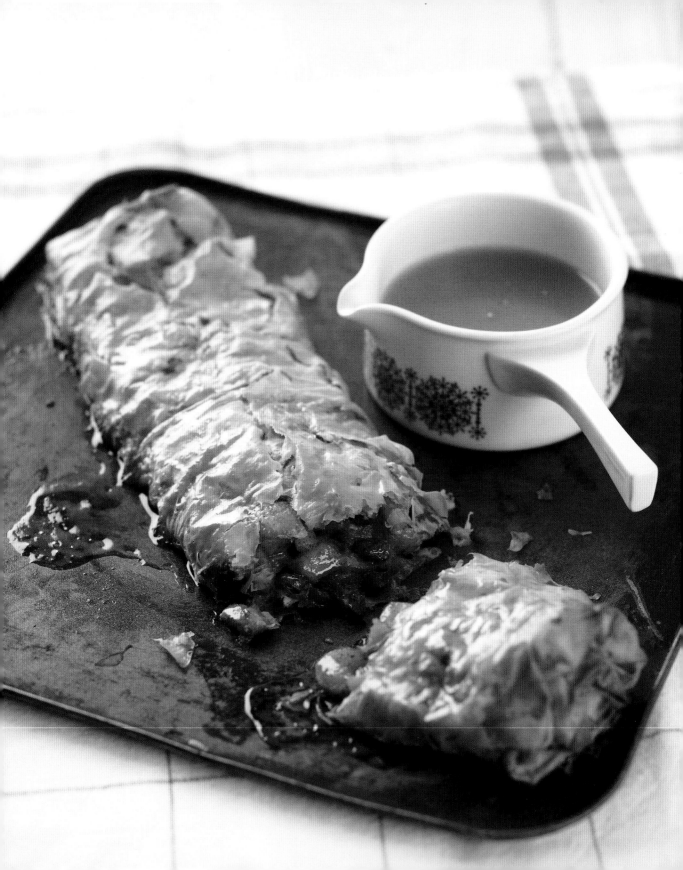

Apple Strudel with 'Cider' Sauce

This dish shows just how easy it is to incorporate lots of fruit servings into a tasty, delectable dessert! Filo pastry is such an easy and healthy alternative to traditional, butter-loaded pastry. Just remember, once opened, keep it covered with a clean, damp tea towel until you are ready to use it, otherwise it will dry out.

SERVES 8

8 eating apples, peeled, cored and finely chopped
1 tbsp lemon juice
115g (4oz) sultanas
1 tsp ground cinnamon
½ tsp ground nutmeg
1 tbsp soft brown sugar (light or dark is fine)
6 sheets filo pastry, thawed and covered with a clean, damp, tea towel
light cooking spray

For the sauce
1 tbsp cornflour
450ml (16fl oz) dry cider or apple juice

1 Preheat the oven to 190°C/375°F/Gas mark 5.

2 Line a baking tray with non-stick baking parchment.

3 Put the apples into a bowl with the lemon juice, sultanas, cinnamon, nutmeg and sugar. Mix together well and set aside.

4 Unroll the pastry, lay out one sheet on the prepared baking sheet and spray it very lightly with cooking spray. Now, place the next sheet on top and spray with cooking spray, then put one more sheet on top. Repeat with the remaining filo. (You will make 2 strudels each using 3 sheets of filo pastry.)

5 Divide the apple mixture between the 2 pastry stacks and spread out evenly, leaving a 5cm (2in) border of pastry at each end. Now, carefully roll the pastry up, lengthways, tucking in the edges as you go. Make sure you finishing rolling with the seam at the bottom, so that the weight of the strudel seals the edge. Spray the strudels lightly with cooking spray and bake for 30 minutes or until crisp and golden.

6 To make the sauce, in a small saucepan, blend the cornflour with the cider or apple juice, then bring to the boil while stirring constantly. Pour the sauce over the strudel and serve while warm.

Chargrilled Fruit

Fruit is an obvious choice when looking for a healthy dessert, and this recipe kicks up the naturally sweet flavours to make a moreish guilt-free dessert, which is perfect served with low-fat fromage frais or with a piece of fat-free cake. This dish works equally well on the barbecue.

SERVES 4

1 pineapple
1 papaya
1 mango
6 tbsp clear honey
grated zest of 1 orange
grated zest of 1 lemon
1 x 2.5cm (1in) piece
   of fresh root ginger,
   peeled and grated
4 kiwi fruit, peeled
   and slices
2 nectarines, peeled
   and halved
2 bananas, peeled
   and halved

TIP
Why not make a smoothie with the remaining fruit? Simply whiz everything up in a blender or liquidiser with a few ice cubes and a fresh orange.

1   Preheat the grill to medium.

2   Peel and core the pineapple, then slice into rings. You will need 4 pineapple rings for this dish, so save the rest of the pineapple for another day.

3   Cut the papaya in half and scoop out the seeds with a spoon. Peel the skin and slice the flesh. Use 4 slices for this recipe and save the rest.

4   Slice the mango in half through to the stone, then twist to remove the flesh from the stone. Again, you will be using 4 slices for this dish.

5   Now, mix the honey, grated orange and lemon zest and grated ginger together in a large bowl and add all the fruit pieces, including the kiwi, nectarines and bananas. Using your fingers, gently move the fruit around to coat in the glaze, then arrange the fruit on a baking tray that will fit neatly under the grill.

6   Cook under the hot grill for 10 minutes, turning frequently and adding extra glaze on each turn. When nicely browned, divide among 4 serving plates and serve immediately.

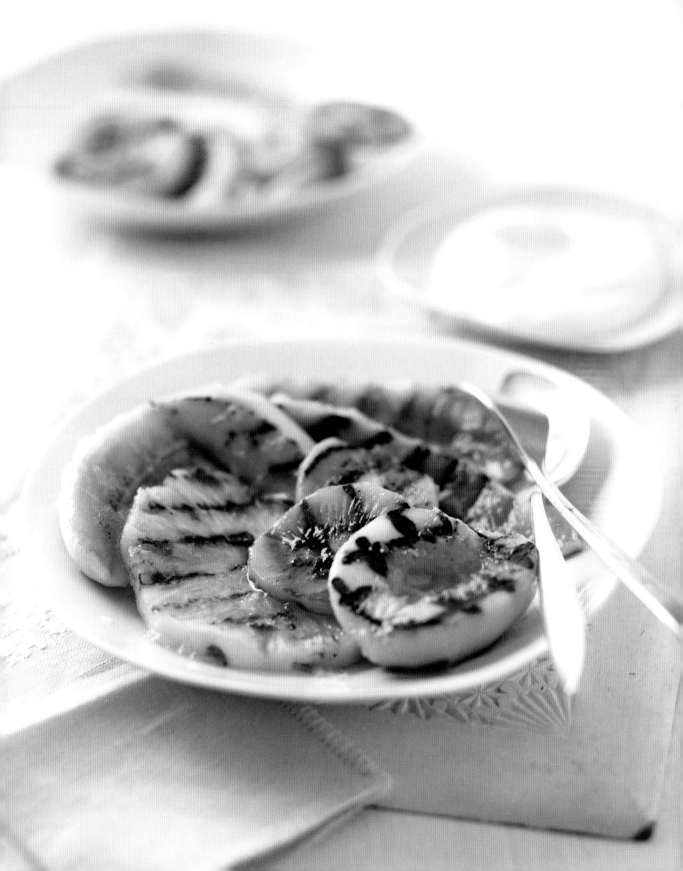

Peach Upside-down Pudding

This is a lightly sweetened cake that allows the fresh flavour of the peaches to shine through. Based on a traditional tarte tatin, having the right pan to cook this in will help with its success, so use either a tarte tatin tin or a skillet, which is a heavy frying pan that you can also put in the oven.

SERVES 6

light cooking spray
  or low-fat spread,
  for coating or greasing
200g (7oz) plain
  wholewheat flour
2 tsp baking powder
1 tsp bicarbonate of soda
1 tsp ground ginger
150g (5½oz) demerara
  sugar
225ml (8fl oz) fat-free
  buttermilk
1 tsp lemon juice
grated zest of ½ lemon
2 tbsp orange juice
620g (1lb 5oz) peeled
  and sliced fresh peaches
  (or canned peaches in
  grape juice)

1 Preheat the oven to 180°C/350°F/Gas mark 4.

2 Spray a 25cm (10in) tarte tatin tin or 'skillet' well with light cooking spray or grease well with low-fat spread.

3 In a medium bowl, combine the wholemeal flour, baking powder, bicarbonate of soda, ginger and 100g (3½oz) of the demerara sugar.

4 In a separate jug, combine the buttermilk, lemon juice and grated zest and mix well.

5 Now, combine the orange juice and the remaining demerara sugar in the tarte tatin tin or skillet.

6 Next, place your tarte tatin tin or skillet over a medium heat and stir continuously until the sugar is completely melted and starting to bubble. Be careful not to let it burn. As soon as it starts to reduce, place the peaches on top of the sugar, trying to fill in all the gaps, then remove from heat and set aside.

7 Next, pour the combined liquid ingredients into the flour mixture, and beat with a wooden spoon until smooth. Now, pour this batter over the peaches, making sure they are completely covered.

recipe continues...

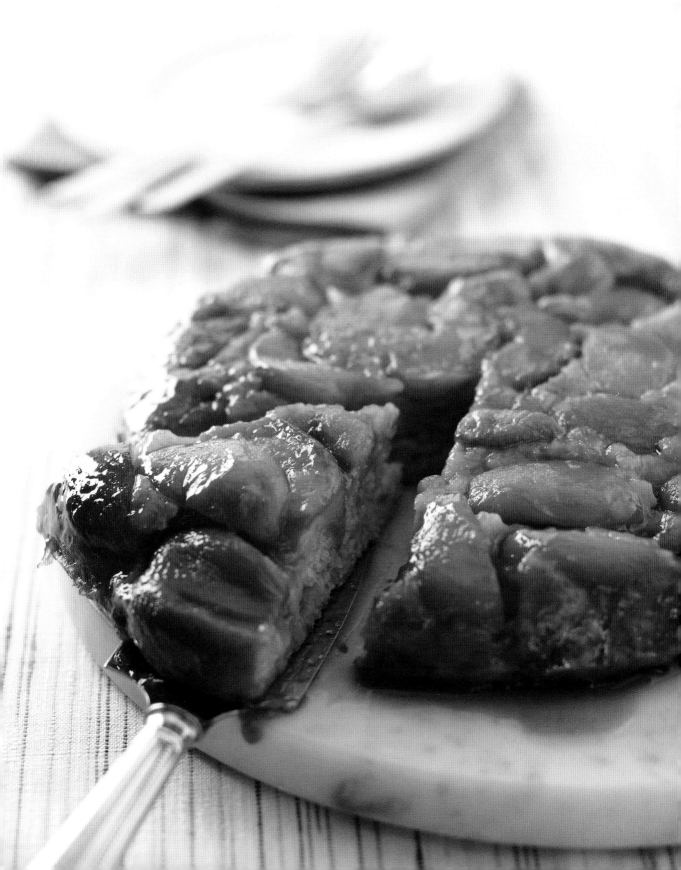

8 Put the tin or skillet into the oven (you may want to place a baking sheet on the shelf below it to catch drips) and bake for 30–40 minutes until the sides of the cake pull away from the edges of the tin and a skewer inserted into the centre of the sponge comes out clean.

9 Remove from the oven and allow to cool in the tin or skillet for about 15–20 minutes.

10 Use a knife to loosen around the edges of the cake; try not to damage the sponge. Once you feel that the cake is loose enough, place a large plate or serving platter over the top and turn the tin or skillet upside down. You might want to do this over the sink in case of drips! Remove the tin or skillet carefully from the cake and scrape out any remaining yummy, scrunchy bits!

Low-fat Hot Bitter Sweet Pudding

This is a delicious and very quick dessert that offers sweetness and bitterness from the coffee. Don't be put off by the cup of coffee you will pour on top of the pudding before you cook it. It will look strange and it is supposed to look like that, but don't worry, it will all soak into the sponge as it cooks and go all gooey at the bottom. Yum! You can make this dessert a day ahead as it keeps well.

SERVES 6

light cooking spray
  or low-fat spread,
  for coating or greasing
150g (5½oz) plain flour
30g (1oz) unsweetened
  cocoa powder
2 tsp baking powder
75g (2½oz) caster sugar
125ml (4fl oz) skimmed
  milk
1 large egg, lightly beaten
2 tbsp light olive oil
1 tsp vanilla extract
75g 2½oz pecan nut halves
80g (3oz) soft brown sugar
225ml (8fl oz) hot coffee

1   Preheat the oven to 190°C/375°F/Gas mark 5.

2   Spray a 20 x 20cm (8 x 8in) baking dish with light cooking spray or grease with low-fat spread.

3   In a large bowl, sift together the flour, cocoa and baking powder, then add the caster sugar.

4   Mix together the milk, beaten egg, olive oil and vanilla extract in jug.

5   Now, make a well in centre of the dry ingredients and gradually pour in the milk mixture, stirring with a wooden spoon until combined.

6   Stir in the pecans, then spoon the mixture into the prepared baking dish and spread evenly. Set aside.

7   Next, dissolve the brown sugar in the hot coffee and gently pour this over the batter. This will look a bit strange because the coffee will just 'float' on top of the batter, but it'll turn out beautifully, I promise!

8   Bake in the oven for about 25 minutes or until a cocktail stick inserted into the centre comes out clean. Leave to stand for 10 minutes before serving straight from the dish.

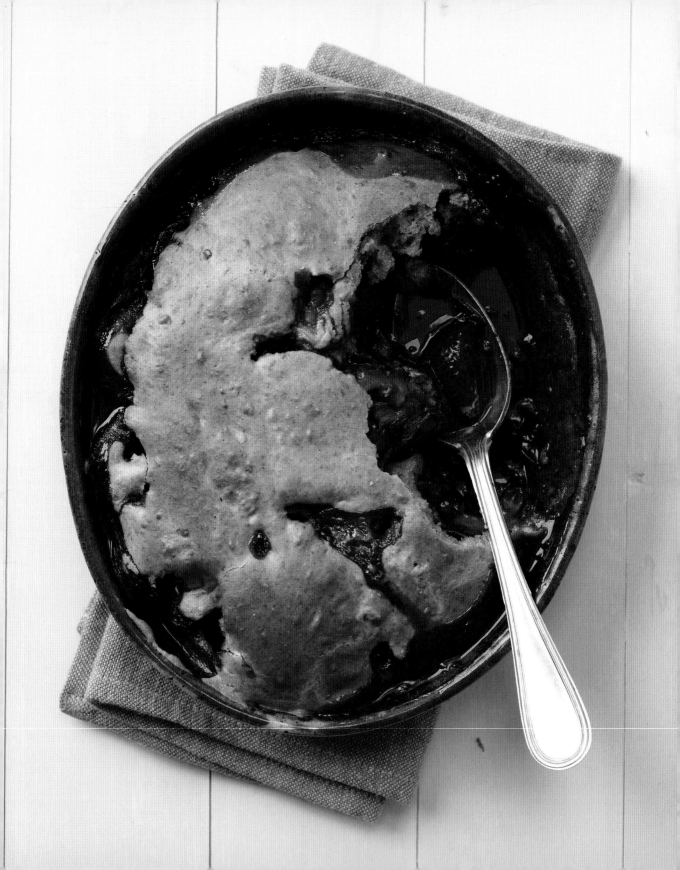

Gingerbread Plum Pudding

Make this pudding when plums are in season and are nice and sweet. Plums and gingerbread are such a great combination – sweet and spicy all in one go.

SERVES 4-6

55g (2oz) low-fat, heart-
  healthy spread,
  plus extra for greasing
675g (1½lb) plums,
  washed, pitted
  and cut in half
175g (6oz) light
  muscovado sugar
1 tbsp good-quality
  maple syrup
1 tbsp golden syrup
5 tbsp skimmed milk
2 eggs, beaten
225g (8oz) plain flour
1 tsp ground mixed spice
1 tsp ground ginger
1 tsp ground cinnamon
1 tsp baking powder

1 Preheat the oven to 180°C/350°F/Gas mark 4.

2 Grease a 1 litre (1¾ pint) ovenproof, shallow dish with a little extra low-fat spread.

3 In a large bowl, mix the plums and the muscovado sugar together. Place the halved plums, cut side facing up, in the bottom of the prepared dish. Sprinkle over any remaining sugar from the bowl and set aside.

4 Next, put the low-fat spread and both syrups into a saucepan and melt over a low heat stirring continuously. Now, add the milk, stir, remove from the heat and set aside for 10 minutes to cool.

5 Once cooled, crack in the eggs and whisk together using a hand whisk.

6 Now, sift the flour, spices and baking powder into the syrup and milk mixture and beat together using a wooden spoon.

7 Pour the gingerbread mix over the plums and spread over evenly covering all the edges. Bake for 45 minutes until the gingerbread is coming away slightly from the edges. Serve hot!

Glazed Apricot Sponge Pudding

Sponge puddings can be very high in saturated fat, but this healthy version uses the minimum of oil, no butter and no eggs. I have used canned apricots here, but this will work just as well with canned peaches or pears.

SERVES 4

2 tbsp sunflower oil,
   plus extra for oiling
2 tsp golden syrup
410g (14½oz) can apricot
   halves in natural juice
150g (5½oz) self-raising
   flour
75g (3oz) fresh wholemeal
   breadcrumbs
90g (3oz) light muscovado
   sugar
1 tsp ground cinnamon
175ml (6fl oz) skimmed milk

1 Preheat the oven to 180°C/350°F/Gas mark 4.

2 Oil a 900ml (1½ pint) pudding basin with a little extra sunflower oil.

3 Start by spooning the golden syrup into the base of the prepared pudding basin.

4 Now, drain the apricots and reserve the juice, then arrange about 8 apricot halves in the pudding basin.

5 Using a food processor or blender, purée the remaining apricots along with the reserved juice from the can and set aside.

6 In a separate bowl, mix the flour, breadcrumbs, muscovado sugar and cinnamon together until combined. Now, beat in the sunflower oil and skimmed milk until nice and smooth.

7 Spoon the mixture on top of the apricots in the basin and bake for 50–55 minutes or until firm and golden.

8 Allow the dessert to cool for 10 minutes before turning out upside down onto a serving plate and serving with the puréed fruit along side.

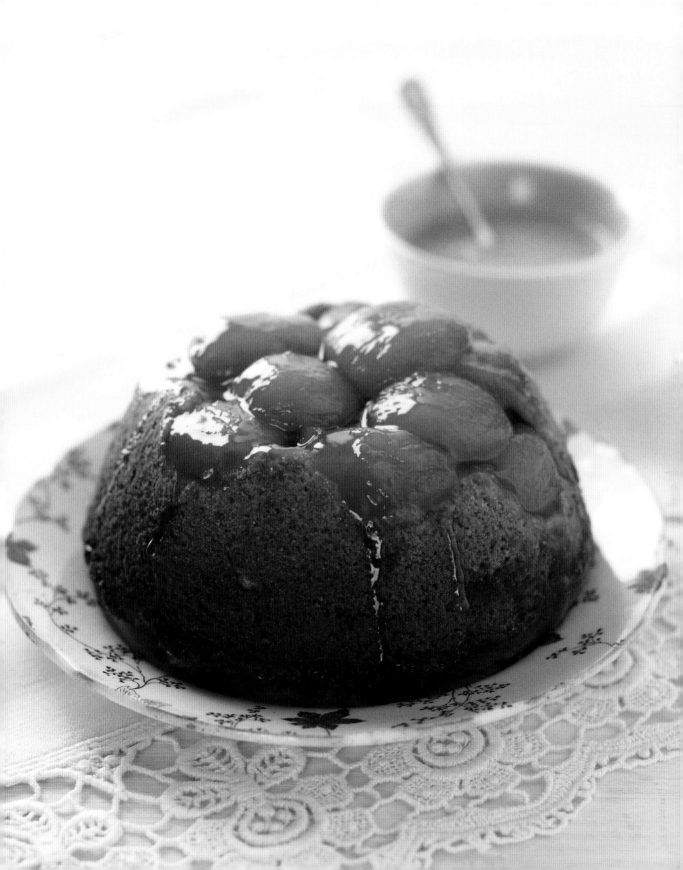

Grilled Peaches with Gingernut Topping

This dessert works equally well done on the barbecue or under a grill. Just make sure it's *hot*! And definitely go with the shop-bought gingernut biscuits – they make this dessert just that little bit extra special.

SERVES 4

300g (10½oz) raspberries
1 vanilla pod, split in half
  lengthways
1 tbsp apple juice
4 just-ripe peaches,
  cut in half and pitted
1 tbsp soft dark brown
  sugar
25g (1oz) gingernut
  biscuits, crushed,
  to serve

TIP
A dollop of low-fat crème fraîche or yogurt goes beautifully with this dish.

1 Preheat the barbecue or grill until very hot.

2 Pop the raspberries, vanilla pod and apple juice into a saucepan and bring to a simmer over a medium heat for 2–3 minutes. Set this mixture aside and allow to cool for a few minutes.

3 Once cooled, remove the vanilla pod and set aside. Push the mixture through a fine metal sieve into a separate bowl to remove all the pips, then put the vanilla pod back into the mixture and chill in the refrigerator until needed.

4 Meanwhile, sprinkle the cut side of the peaches with the soft brown sugar and put on the barbecue or under the grill for 2 minutes until lightly charred and softened.

5 Serve with a drizzle of the raspberry sauce and a scattering of the crushed biscuits.

Juicy Berry Cobbler

Juicy is the right word for this pudding. I think I would like it cold the next day, but there has never been any left to put that to the test! Don't worry about using frozen fruit – it retains the majority of the goodness and means that you can always have some ready for action in the freezer.

SERVES 8

light cooking spray
  or low-fat spread,
  for coating or greasing
3 tbsp soft brown sugar
2 tbsp cornflour
60ml (2fl oz) plus 2 tbsp
  orange juice
1kg (2¼lb) fresh
  or frozen cherries,
  blueberries,
  blackberries, etc

For the cobbler
100g (3½oz) wholemeal
  plain flour
30g (1oz) wheat bran
70g (2½oz) caster sugar
1½ tsp baking powder
½ tsp bicarbonate of soda
175ml (6fl oz) low-fat
  buttermilk

1   Preheat the oven to 180°C/350°F/Gas mark 4.

2   Spray or grease a 2 litre (3½ pint) casserole dish with light cooking spray or low-fat spread.

3   To make the fruit filling, put the brown sugar, cornflour and orange juice in a medium, non-stick saucepan and stir well. Add the fruit and cook over a medium heat, stirring constantly, for about 5 minutes until the mixture is thick and bubbling. Pour the cooked fruit mixture into the casserole dish and set aside.

4   To make the cobbler topping, in a large bowl, combine the flour, wheat bran, caster sugar, baking powder and bicarbonate of soda. Now, add the buttermilk and, using a wooden spoon, mix until smooth. Pour the batter over the fruit and bake for about 30 minutes or until golden brown and bubbling.

Healthy Bread & Butter Pudding

For those who love old-fashioned 'nursery' puddings, this is for you – but a bit healthier than the traditional version. Wholemeal bread, low-fat heart-healthy spread and skimmed milk won't put you on the naughty step.

SERVES 6

40g (1½oz) low-fat, heart-
  healthy spread,
  plus extra for greasing
12 slices brown or
  wholemeal bread,
  crusts cut off
  (medium thickness)
900ml (1½ pints) semi-
  skimmed milk
½ tsp vanilla extract
8 egg yolks
175g (6oz) caster sugar
25g (1oz) raisins
25g (1oz) sultanas
fresh nutmeg, to grate
2 tbsp soft brown sugar
  to caramelise on top

1 Preheat the oven to 180°C/350°F/Gas mark 4.

2 Lightly grease a 1 x 1.5 litre (2½ pint) pudding dish or basin with low-fat spread.

3 Spread the sliced brown bread with low-fat spread and set aside.

4 In a saucepan, heat the milk with the vanilla extract and bring to the boil, then remove from the heat and set aside.

5 While the milk is cooling a little, whisk together the egg yolks and caster sugar in a bowl. Now, strain the warm milk onto the egg yolks and sugar. Bingo – you've just made custard!

6 Cut the bread into triangular halves, and begin arranging in the prepared dish in layers. Between each layer, sprinkle with the raisins and sultanas and a grating of fresh nutmeg. On the last layer, and around the edge, position the slices of bread with pointy bits sticking up, as these will brown and caramelise, and be delicious.

7 Next, pour over the warm custard, lightly pressing the bread to help it soak in and leave to stand for at least 20–30 minutes.

recipe continues...

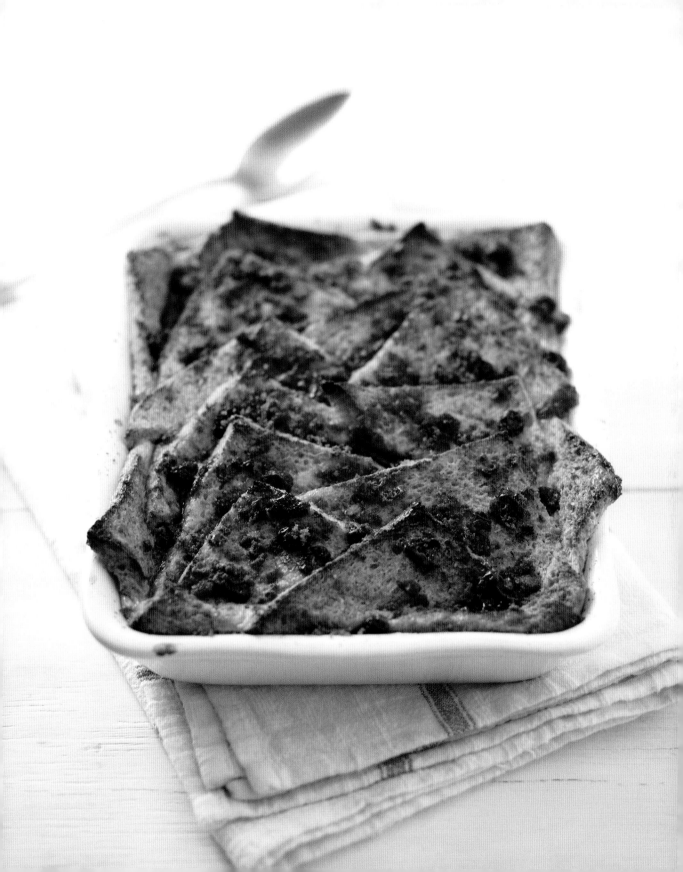

8 Bake for 20–30 minutes until the pudding begins to set. Don't overcook it, or the custard will scramble. Remove from the oven and sprinkle with the soft brown sugar. Preheat the grill.

9 Next, put under a hot grill to caramelise for about 5 minutes or until nicely brown with a crunchy, golden finish.

Sticky Figs with Pistachios

Fresh figs are sweet and flavoursome, and this dish not only looks beautiful, it also tastes sensational. You can serve this either as a dessert or a late afternoon treat with friends.

SERVES 4

8 ripe figs
4 tbsp clear honey
1 tbsp soft dark
  brown sugar
1 tsp ground mixed spice
55g (2oz) unsalted
  pistachio nuts, chopped
low-fat fromage frais,
  to serve

1 Preheat the grill to medium.

2 Cut a criss-cross across the top of the figs, so that they open out like a flower and you can squeeze the middle to loosen.

3 Put the opened figs in a shallow baking dish and drizzle over the honey. Sprinkle over the sugar, mixed spice and chopped pistachios.

4 Pop under the grill for 5–6 minutes until warmed through and the honey has melted to the bottom. Serve warm with low-fat fromage frais on the side.

Light Banana Rice Pudding

Rice puddings always used to be a little thick and heavy, but by adding whisked egg whites this dessert is so light that it almost floats away!

SERVES 6

low-fat spread,
  for greasing
60g (2¼oz) short-grain
  pudding rice
600ml (1 pint) semi-
  skimmed milk
3 tbsp clear honey
1 vanilla pod, split
  in half lengthways
2 ripe bananas
finely grated zest
  of ½ lemon
2 egg whites
a pinch of freshly grated
  nutmeg or ½ tsp ground
  nutmeg

TIP
You can freeze ripe bananas until you are ready to use them. If you have some bananas that are perfectly ripe but you don't have any plans for them, simply peel them, then pop in a freezer bag and freeze until you are ready to use them.

1   Grease six 200ml (7fl oz) ramekins with a little low-fat spread.

2   Place the rice in a non-stick lidded saucepan. Pour in the milk, then stir in the honey and add the vanilla pod. Over a medium heat, bring gently to the boil, then reduce the heat and cover with the lid.

3   Simmer for 1 hour–1 hour 15 minutes, stirring occasionally to prevent it sticking, until the rice is soft and the mixture has thickened but is still sloppy.

4   Meanwhile, heat the oven to 200°C/400°F/Gas Mark 6.

5   Remove the vanilla pod from the rice. Peel the bananas and slice them thinly, then fold them into the rice with the grated lemon zest.

6   Using a free-standing electric mixer, whisk the egg whites until soft peaks form. Gently fold them into the rice mixture with a large metal spoon. Now, spoon the mixture it into the prepared ramekins and sprinkle the top with the nutmeg.

7   Place the ramekins on a baking sheet and bake for 10–12 minutes until golden brown and well risen. Serve warm.

Hot Choccy Soufflé

If you want to impress a loved one – serve them this simple chocolate soufflé!
Don't be afraid if you've never made a soufflé before, it's pretty easy really!

SERVES 2

tiny knob of softened
  butter, for greasing
25g (1oz) caster sugar,
  plus 3 tsp
50g (1¾oz) good-quality
  plain dark chocolate (at
  least 70% cocoa solids),
  broken into small pieces
2 eggs, separated
cocoa powder, for dusting

1 Preheat the oven to 200°C/400°F/Gas mark 6.

2 Place a baking tray in the oven to warm. Make sure
   you leave enough space between the oven racks for
   the soufflés to rise.

3 Rub the knob of butter around the inside of
   2 ramekins, then add 1 teaspoon of caster sugar to
   each ramekin and swirl it around so that the butter is
   covered with a thin layer of sugar. Shake off any sugar
   that hasn't stuck.

4 Now, place the chocolate in a large heatproof bowl
   set over a pan of simmering water and melt, stirring
   continuously. Remove from the heat.

5 Meanwhile, mix the egg yolks with 25g (1oz) caster
   sugar together in a bowl with a wooden spoon until
   it becomes creamy. Stir the yolk mixture into the
   melted chocolate.

6 Using a free-standing electric mixer, whisk the egg
   whites until they begin to form stiff peaks. Now, add
   the remaining teaspoon of sugar and keep whisking
   until it is stiff and shiny and glossy.

7 Stir a spoonful of the whites into the bowl of
   chocolate and stir gently to loosen the mix. Carefully
   fold in the rest of the egg whites using a large metal
   spoon or spatula.

8 Spoon the soufflé mix into the prepared ramekins and
   bake for about 10 minutes when they should have
   risen but still have a little wobble in the middle. When
   the soufflés are ready, remove them from the oven
   and put onto a serving plate. Dust with cocoa powder
   and serve immediately.

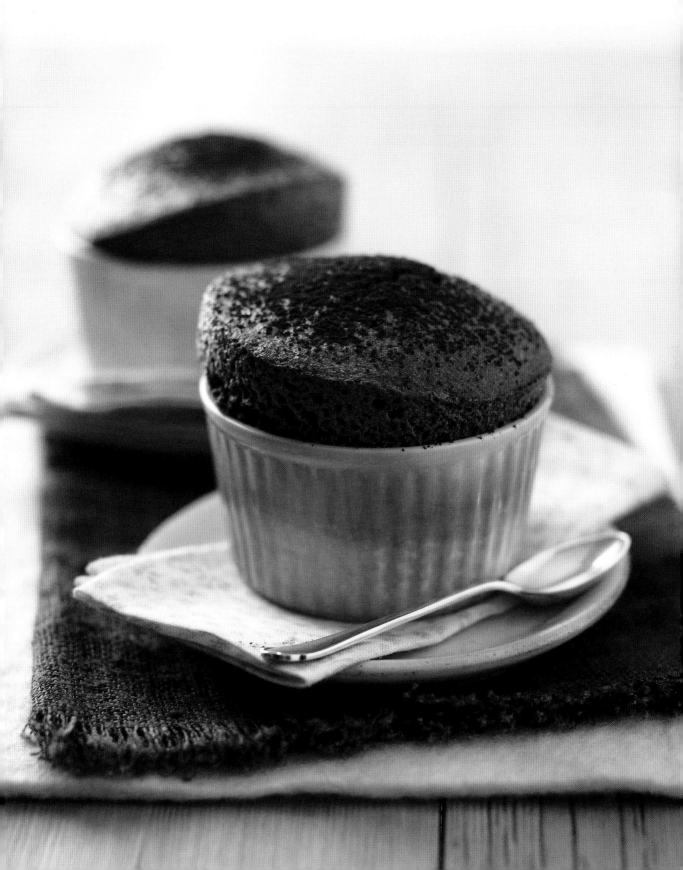

Fruit & Nut Roast

Ah, this is a real treat that could be eaten everyday, full of goodness and flavour! Follow the recipe, but also feel free to add anything else you think might work.

SERVES 6

3-4 (about 500g/1lb 2oz) peaches, quartered and pitted
3-4 (about 300g/10½oz) plums, halved and pitted
1 vanilla pod, split lengthways
large pinch of saffron strands
150ml (5fl oz) pomegranate juice
50g (1¾oz) blueberries
50g (1¾oz) raspberries
25g (1oz) barley flakes
50g (1¾oz) chopped nuts, such as hazelnuts, pistachios, pecan nuts, walnuts, etc
2 tbsp demerara sugar

1 Preheat the oven to 190°C/375°F/Gas mark 5.

2 Arrange the peaches and plums in a single layer in a large baking dish. Add the 2 halves of the vanilla pod, the saffron and the pomegranate juice and bake, uncovered, for 30 minutes until tender. Switch off the oven.

3 Now, add the blueberries and raspberries to the baking dish and return to the oven and warm for a further 10 minutes. Remove from the oven and set aside to cool slightly.

4 Meanwhile, toast the barley flakes and the chopped nuts in a non-stick frying pan over a medium heat until lightly golden.

5 Sprinkle the demerara sugar over the nuts and flakes and allow to melt. Stir well, then sprinkle over the roasted fruit and serve at once.

Plum Tarte Tatin

This recipe uses shop-bought puff pastry, so try to look for the 'light' pastry, as this contains only half the fat. Also make sure you use very firm plums. If they are too ripe and soft, they will produce too much juice and drown the pastry! This is a dish that often looks messy, but just close your eyes and enjoy the delicious taste! You will need an 28cm (11in) tarte tatin tin or 'skillet' for this dish.

SERVES 6

25g (1oz) low-fat, heart-healthy spread
25g (1oz) golden caster sugar
800g (1lb 12oz) firm plums, halved and pitted
55g (2oz) ground almonds
500g (1lb 2oz) packet frozen 'light' puff pastry, thawed
plain flour, for dusting
low-fat fromage frais, to serve

1 Preheat the oven to 200°C/400°F/Gas mark 6.

2 Melt the low-fat spread in the tarte tatin tin or 'skillet' over a medium heat. Add the sugar and 1 tablespoon of water and stir for 2–3 minutes until browned. Remove from the heat and place the plums, cut side up, in the tin.

3 Sprinkle the ground almonds evenly over the plums.

4 Roll out the pastry (unless it is ready rolled) on a lightly floured surface until it is 4cm (1½in) larger than the tin or skillet, all the way around. Lift the pastry into the tin and tuck it down in between the plums and the inside edge of the tin.

5 Bake for 30–35 minutes until the pastry has risen and is nice and crispy. Allow to cool in the tin or skillet for 10 minutes, then turn out onto a large plate. Be very careful: I suggest you do this over the sink, as some hot juices may pour out. Serve with low-fat fromage frais.

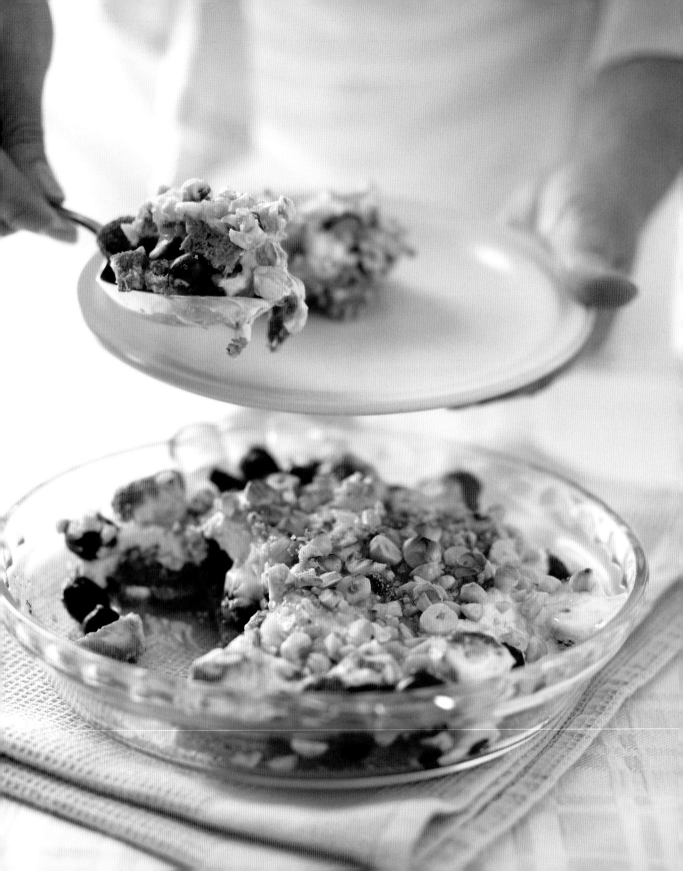

Nearly Summer Pudding

This is a summer pudding with a twist. It is very simple to make and is best served hot – this is one of my favourites!

low-fat spread,
  for greasing
4 slices of brown or
  wholemeal bread,
  crusts cut off
4 tbsp demerara sugar
2 tsp cornflour
200g (7oz) low-fat
  fromage frais
275g (10oz) mixed fresh
  summer berries or
  frozen summer berry
  mix, such as raspberries,
  blueberries, strawberries,
  redcurrants, etc
85g (3oz) chopped
  hazelnuts

1 Preheat the grill to high.

2 Grease a 23cm (9in) round or equivalent size pie dish with a little low-fat spread.

3 Arrange the slices of bread on the base of the dish and sprinkle with 2 tablespoons of demerara sugar. Pop under the hot grill to toast and caramelise for 3–4 minutes.

4 Meanwhile, in a small bowl, mix the cornflour and fromage frais together, then set aside.

5 Once the bread has been grilled until crispy and caramelised, remove from the grill and cover with the fruit, leaving the edges of the bread exposed.

6 Now, dollop the fromage frais mixture over the fruit, sprinkle with the final 2 tablespoons of sugar and the chopped hazelnuts.

7 Pop back under the grill, as close to the top as you can and grill for 6–8 minutes until everything is starting to bubble and brown.

Passionate Pear Crumble

I've called this 'passionate' because it's perfect to share with loved ones. With just a tiny bit of butter, lots of fruit and a high-fibre topping, this pear crumble will quickly become a family favourite.

SERVES 6-8

40g (1½oz) low-fat, heart-healthy spread, plus extra for greasing
8 ripe Conference pears, peeled, cored and sliced
grated zest of 1 lemon
grated zest of 1 orange
2 tbsp golden caster sugar
½ tsp grated nutmeg
25g (1oz) skimmed milk powder
25g (1oz) ground almonds
50g (1¾oz) porridge oats
175g (6oz) wholemeal plain flour
110g (4oz) soft dark brown sugar
1 tsp ground cinnamon
low-fat custard or low-fat crème fraîche, to serve

1 Preheat the oven to 200°C/400°F/Gas mark 6.

2 Grease a 2 litre (3½ pint) pudding dish with a little extra low-fat spread.

3 Place the sliced pears, citrus zest, caster sugar, nutmeg and 100ml (3½fl oz) water in the base of the baking dish.

4 In a large bowl, combine all the dry ingredients together, add the low-fat spread and, using your fingertips, rub it in quickly (before the spread melts in the heat of your hands) until the mixture resembles breadcrumbs.

5 Loosely spread the crumble mixture on top of the pears and bake for 45 minutes–1 hour or until the top is golden. Serve warm with low-fat custard or low-fat crème fraîche.

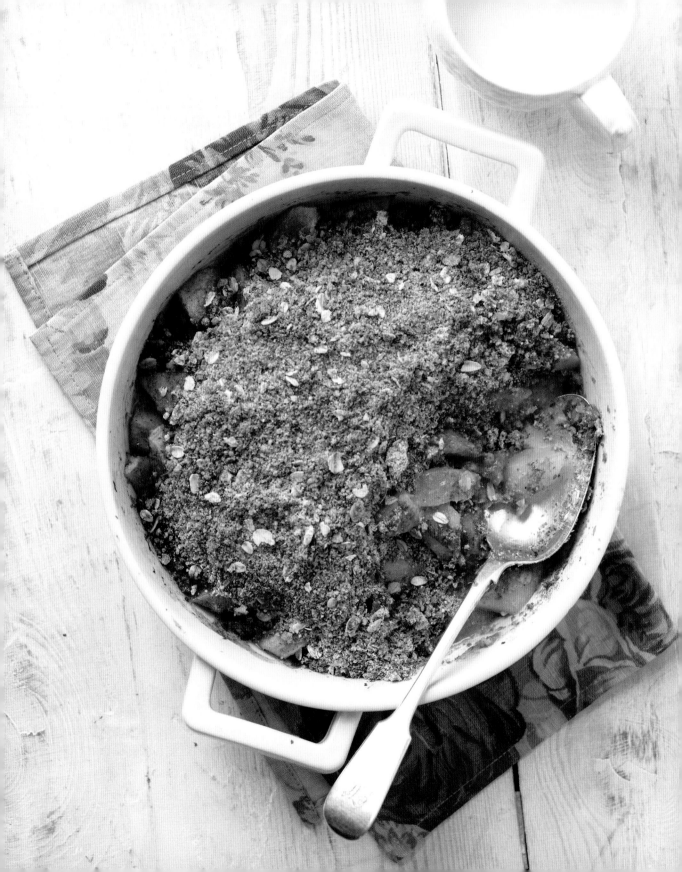

Red Berry Superfood Crumble

The benefit is in the title – superfood! Dark red berries are packed full of nutrients for a healthy heart, so this is just what the doctor ordered. If using frozen fruit, thaw before using.

SERVES 8

500g mixed berries,
  such as raspberries,
  redcurrants and
  blackberries
55g (2oz) low-fat,
  heart-healthy spread
90g (3oz) wholemeal flour
60g (2¼oz) demerara
  sugar
½ tsp ground cinnamon
50g (1¾oz) flaked almonds
50g (1¾oz) chopped
  walnuts or pecan nuts
low-fat crème fraîche,
  to serve

1 Preheat the oven to 180°C/350°F/Gas mark 4.

2 Put the berries straight into an ovenproof pie dish. No need to grease this beforehand.

3 In a large mixing bowl, rub the low-fat spread into the flour, squashing it through your fingertips to form breadcrumbs. Stir through the sugar, cinnamon, almonds and chopped nuts.

4 Spoon the crumble mixture over the berries and bake for 25 minutes or until golden and bubbling. Simple as that! Serve with low-fat crème fraîche.

Redcurrant & Peach Sponge Delight

Such a lovely combination of flavours that still manages to be relatively fat-free, this pudding is very simple to make, so much so that I let the children loose on this one while I put my feet up!

SERVES 10

low-fat spread,
  for greasing
150g (5½oz) Quark
  (virtually fat-free soft
  cheese)
3 tbsp skimmed milk
3 tbsp sunflower oil
2 eggs
75g (2½oz) golden caster
  sugar, plus 1 tbsp
250g (9oz) self-raising flour
grated zest of 2 oranges
100g (3½oz) redcurrants
  (or you could use
  blueberries)
3–4 ripe peaches,
  pitted and sliced

1 Preheat the oven to 180°C/350°F/Gas mark 4.

2 Grease a loose-bottomed 23cm (9in) round cake tin with low-fat spread and line the base non-stick baking parchment.

3 Place the Quark, milk, sunflower oil, eggs and 75g (2½oz) sugar in a large bowl and, using a wooden spoon, beat together until smooth.

4 Now, sift in the flour and add the grated orange zest and half of the redcurrants. Fold all of these ingredients in carefully using a spatula. Pour the mixture into the prepared cake tin.

5 Place the sliced peaches and the remaining redcurrants on top of the mixture and sprinkle with the extra tablespoon of sugar. Bake for 45 minutes until golden brown.

6 Allow to cool in the tin for 10 minutes, then turn out onto a serving plate, remove the paper and serve warm or cold.

Apples in Red Wine

Red wine is considered great for your heart as long as it's taken in moderation. So when mixed with apples and antioxidant-packed raspberries, this dish can be eaten guilt-free. Antioxidants are thought to cut our risk of heart disease and certain cancers and the general rule is: the deeper the colour, the more antioxidant-rich the food. Therefore, raspberries not only taste delicious, but are packed with goodness.

SERVES 2

4 eating apples, peeled,
  cored and cut into
  thick wedges
2 tbsp lemon juice
40g (1½oz) low-fat, heart-
  healthy spread
55g (2oz) light muscovado
  sugar
1 small orange
1 cinnamon stick, broken
150ml (5fl oz) red wine
225g (8oz) raspberries,
  hulled and thawed
  if frozen
fresh mint sprigs,
  to decorate

TIP
This dessert makes a lovely accompaniment to the German Honey Cake on page 36.

1 Place the apples in a bowl and toss in the lemon juice to prevent discolouring.

2 In a non-stick frying pan, melt the low-fat spread over a low heat, then add the sugar and stir to form a paste.

3 Now, stir in the apple wedges and cook for 2 minutes until they are covered in the sugar paste.

4 Using a vegetable peeler, pare off a few strips of orange rind and add to the frying pan with the cinnamon pieces.

5 Now, cut the orange in half and squeeze the juice into the pan along with the red wine. Bring the mixture to the boil, then reduce the heat and simmer gently for 10 minutes. You'll need to watch over this and stir constantly to ensure it doesn't burn.

6 Now, add the raspberries and cook for a further 5 minutes or until the apples are tender. Discard the orange rind and cinnamon pieces, transfer the apple and raspberry mixture to a serving dish, pour all the juices over the top and serve decorated with mint sprigs.

ICES & SORBETS

Blackcurrant Bombes

Packed full of vitamin C, these easy and fun ice lollies will make a healthy change to shop-bought lollies. In my experience, adults love a lolly just as much as the kids do.

MAKES 12 LOLLIES
DEPENDING ON THE MOULD SIZE

200g (7oz) fresh
  blackcurrants
100g (3½oz) caster sugar
grated zest and juice of
  1 unwaxed lemon
300ml (10fl oz) orange
  juice

1 Place the blackcurrants, sugar, lemon zest and lemon juice in a heavy-based pan with 75ml (3fl oz) water. Over a medium heat, dissolve the sugar and then bring to the boil.

2 Reduce the heat and simmer gently for 5 minutes, then remove from the heat and allow to cool.

3 Once cool, blend the mixture with a hand-held electric blender or in a blender or liquidiser until smooth.

4 Now, stir in the orange juice. Tip the mixture into a jug, then pour into lolly moulds and freeze for at least 4 hours until solid.

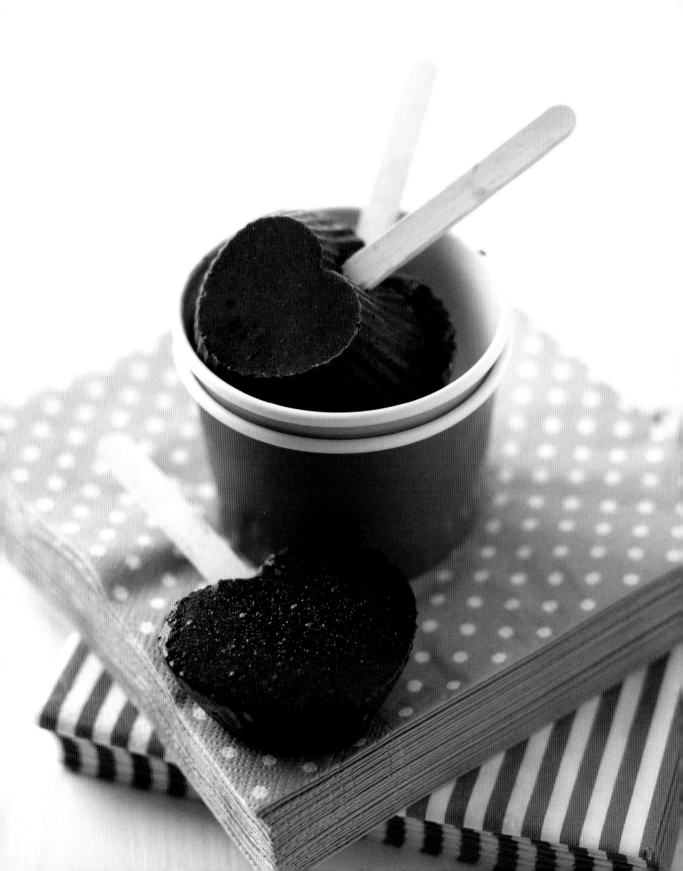

Guava & Agave Lovelies

This is a gorgeous creamy yogurt ice with fresh and funky flavours. I like to freeze the mixture in ice-cube trays to make little blocks. If you have some fun-shaped ice-cube trays, now is the time to dig them out and put them to good use. Guava juice is available in most high street supermarkets, but make sure you buy it unsweetened. Agave nectar is available in most health food shops and is a natural sweetener containing mainly fruit sugar (fructose).

MAKES 2 OR 3 TRAYS OF CUBES
DEPENDING ON YOUR MOULD SIZES

720ml (just under 1¼ pints) unsweetened guava juice
40ml (1½fl oz) low-fat or fat-free vanilla yogurt
1 tbsp lime juice
1 tsp finely grated lime zest
125ml (4fl oz) agave nectar

1 Very simply place all the ingredients in a large bowl and mix together well.

2 Decant the mixture into ice-cube trays or lollipop moulds and freeze for at least 4 hours or until solid.

Classic Lemon Sorbet

Although fat-free, sorbets do contain high quantities of sugar. Having said that, a small portion after a heavy meal will refresh your palate and give you a delightful zing! Ideally you'll need to use an ice-cream maker for this recipe, although you can freeze the mixture in a plastic container and keep stirring it with a fork to break up the ice crystals throughout the freezing process.

**MAKES 750ML
(1¼ PINTS)**

500g (1lb 2oz) caster sugar
**250ml (9fl oz) lemon juice
  (about 6–8 lemons)**
**grated zest of
  1 unwaxed lemon**
**few strands of lemon zest,
  to decorate**

TIP
If you are not using an ice-cream machine: prepare the ingredients in the same way, then pour into a suitable plastic freezerproof container with a lid. Once cooled to room temperature, place in the freezer and check after the first 2 hours and then every hour. Each time you check it, crunch up the forming ice with a fork, then return straight to the freezer. Once completely frozen and set, let the sorbet soften, but not defrost, in the refrigerator for 20 minutes before serving.

1   Put the sugar in a large pan with 750ml (1¼ pints) water and heat gently until the sugar dissolves, then simmer for a couple more minutes.

2   Stir in the lemon juice and grated zest, then allow to cool.

3   Once cool, churn the mixture in an ice-cream machine to sorbet consistency.

4   Serve in scoops, sprinkled with a few strands of lemon zest to decorate.

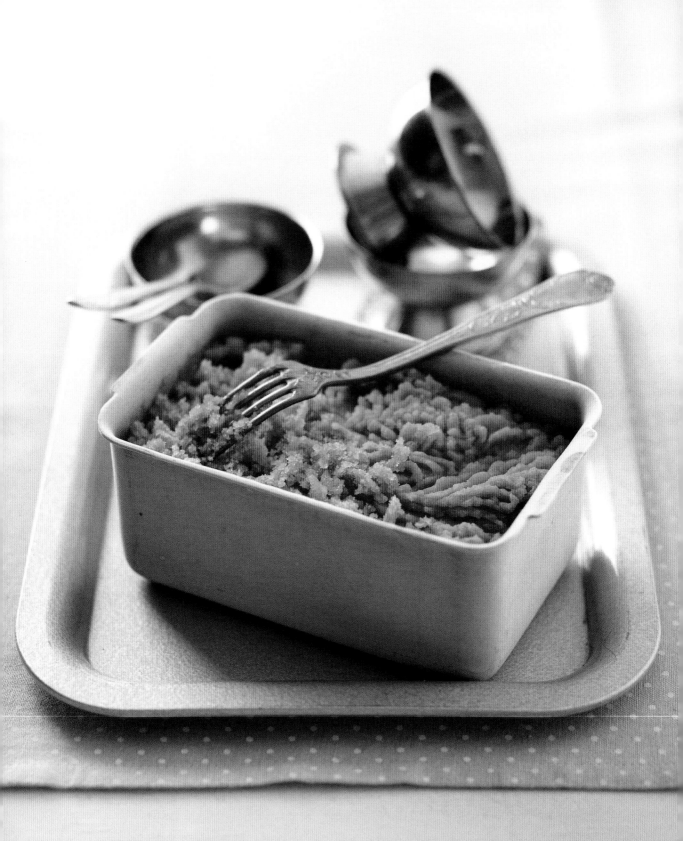

Frozen Melon Granita

This granita equally works well with either watermelon or honeydew melon. If using watermelon, try to get all the seeds out first! Very quick and easy to make, this dessert is a lovely fresh accompaniment to other heavier puddings.

SERVES 4

1 whole small or
  ½ large melon,
  cut into cubes
6 tbsp grape juice
115g (4oz) caster sugar

1   Place all of the ingredients in a food processor and process until smooth.

2   Pour the mixture into a suitable plastic container and freeze for about 1 hour or until frozen and icy around the edges.

3   Remove from the freezer and, using a fork, scrape into light shavings, then stir the ice crystals back into the middle of the dish. Squash any big lumps with the fork.

4   Return to the freezer and repeat the scraping process every hour or so for about 3 hours or until the mixture is icy and granular.

5   When ready to serve, give a final scrape with a fork and serve in individual glasses.

Ginger, Mango & Orange 'Zorbit'

Ah – my taste buds are tingling at the very thought of this one! This sorbet – or, as my friend Anna calls it, 'Zorbit' – is wonderfully refreshing and jam-packed with vitamin C. As it is made from of lots of juice, you'll need an ice-cream maker for this recipe, otherwise it tends to go too solid.

SERVES 8

300g (10½oz) caster sugar
1 x 5cm (2in) piece fresh
  ginger, peeled and
  thinly sliced
grated zest of ½ lime
475ml (16fl oz) orange
  juice
250ml (9fl oz) mango juice
75ml (3fl oz) lemon juice

1 Combine 350ml (12fl oz) water with the sugar, ginger and grated lime zest in a saucepan and bring to the boil. Reduce the heat and simmer for 5 minutes.

2 Allow the mixture to cool, then pass through a sieve.

3 Now, stir in the orange juice, mango juice and lemon juice. Cover and chill for a couple of hours in the refrigerator.

4 Transfer the mixture to an ice-cream maker and freeze according to the manufacturer's instructions. You can serve directly from the ice-cream maker or you can freeze in a suitable plastic container with a lid.

Peach & Cardamom Frozen Yogurt

Low-fat dairy is important to everyone's diet and it has been proven to be beneficial for all of us to have some dairy in our diet everyday – as long as it is the low-fat variety. The peach and cardamom combination will ensure that this very quickly becomes a firm family favourite.

SERVES 4

8 cardamom pods
6 peaches weighing approx 500g (1lb 2oz), halved and pitted
200 ml (7 fl oz) plain low-fat yogurt

1 Crush the cardamom pods using a pestle and mortar or the base of a ramekin.

2 Chop the peaches into small cubes and put them in a lidded saucepan along with the crushed cardamom pods and 2 tablespoons of water. Cover with a lid and simmer gently for about 10 minutes or until the fruit is tender. Remove from the heat and allow to cool.

3 Once cooled, pour the peach mixture into a food processor and blend until smooth. Now, press through a sieve placed over a clean bowl.

4 Add the yogurt to the sieved purée and mix together well. Pour into a suitable plastic freezerproof container with a lid and freeze for about 6 hours until firm, beating with a fork every couple of hours to break up the ice crystals.

5 To serve, remove from the freezer 10 minutes before eating and spoon the yogurt out into small scoops.

Lemon & Lavender Frozen Yogurt

Lemons are rich in vitamin C and are thought to strengthen our immune systems, so this creamy low-fat frozen yogurt makes the most of the delicious and fresh lemon flavour mixed with the calming lavender. Ideally you'll need to use an ice-cream maker for this dish.

SERVES 4

**4 fresh lavender sprigs,
  washed or ½ tsp dried
  lavender**
**720ml (just under 1¼ pints)
  fat-free Greek yogurt**
grated zest of 1 lemon
120ml (4fl oz) lemon juice
180ml (6½fl oz) runny honey

1   If you are using fresh lavender flowers, wash them well and break up using your fingers, discarding the middle stalk.

2   Put the lavender in a bowl with all the other ingredients and mix together with a wooden spoon. Once combined, put the mixture into an ice-cream maker and freeze following the manufacturer's instructions.

3   If you don't have an ice-cream maker, follow the method to combine all the ingredients, then pour into a suitable plastic freezerproof container with a lid and freeze for 2 hours. Remove from the freezer and mix with a fork to break up any lumps, then return to the freezer and freeze for about 6 hours until firm, beating with a fork every couple of hours to break up the ice crystals.

4   Remove from the freezer 15 minutes before serving.

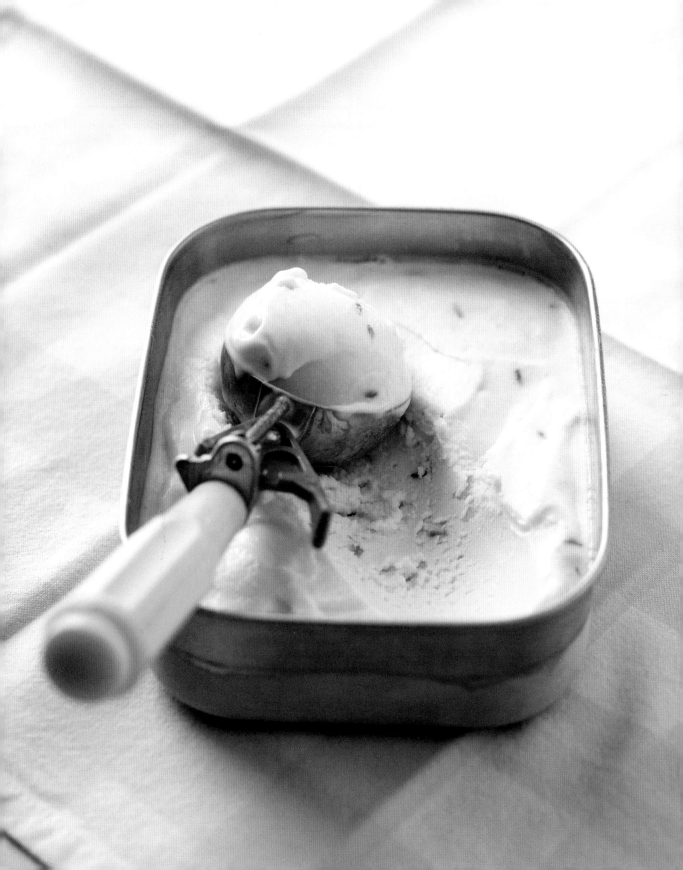

Peach & Strawberry Sorbet

You can use an ice-cream maker for this recipe if you have one or simply freeze in a plastic container and scoop in thin shavings straight onto the plate. This is a deliciously gentle flavour that just tickles the taste buds.

SERVES 4

350g (12oz) sliced fresh
  peaches
150g (5½oz) fresh
  strawberries, hulled
250ml (9fl oz) orange juice
4 tbsp soft dark brown
  sugar

1   Using a food processor, purée the fruit with the orange juice and brown sugar until smooth.

2   Pour the mixture into an ice-cream maker and freeze according to the manufacturer's instructions until firm. You can then serve straight away from the ice-cream maker or freeze for another time in a suitable plastic freezerproof container.

3   If you don't have an ice-cream maker, simply put the mixture into a plastic freezerproof container with a lid and freeze for 6 hours until firm, mashing up any lumps with a fork every couple of hours.

4   Remove from the freezer 10 minutes before serving.

Raspberry & Coconut Ice Pops

Healthy and refreshing on a hot sunny day, these ice pops are perfectly healthy for the children to enjoy. I love making my own ice lollies for the children, and it gives me great peace of mind seeing them enjoy something so much that isn't packed with horrible chemicals and colourings.

MAKES 10-12
DEPENDING ON YOUR MOULD SIZE

150g (5½oz) raspberries
 fresh or frozen
4 tbsp icing sugar
450g (1lb) coconut
 flavoured low-fat
 Greek-style yogurt

1   Using a food processor, purée the raspberries with the icing sugar, then push through a sieve to remove the seeds.

2   Now, spoon half the coconut yogurt into a bowl and stir in 2 tablespoons of the purée so it is coloured pink and streaky.

3   Spoon this mix into the lolly moulds, filling one-third of the way up, then add the rest of the purée and then the rest of the yogurt. Push in lolly sticks and freeze for at least 3 hours until solid.

Rocket Lollies

I remember rocket lollies being my all-time great as a child. I think my kids will have the same memories of these lollies – and I'm very happy about that particularly because these are 100 per cent natural and healthy. You'll need a 12 lolly mould set for this recipe.

MAKES 12 ICE LOLLIES

250g (9oz) strawberries
4 tbsp clear, runny honey
3 large ripe juicy peaches, peeled, pitted and sliced or 1x 450g (16oz) can peaches in juice
5 large ripe kiwi fruit, peeled and sliced

1   Using a blender or liquidiser, purée the strawberries, then push through a sieve to remove the seeds.

2   Stir 2 tablespoons of the honey into the strawberry purée and pour the strawberry mixture into 12 ice lolly moulds until each mould is one-third full. Freeze for 1½–2 hours or until firm.

3   Now, repeat the blending process for the peaches, although there is no need to push them through the sieve. If you are using canned peaches, don't use the juice for this recipe. There is also no need to add any honey to the peach mixture, as they are sweet enough.

4   Pour the mixture into the lolly moulds and freeze for 2 hours.

5   Finally, do the same with the kiwi fruits. These you will need to push through a sieve, then add the remaining honey. Add the kiwi fruit mixture to the lolly moulds and insert lollipop sticks. Freeze for the final time for about 1½–2 hours and enjoy!

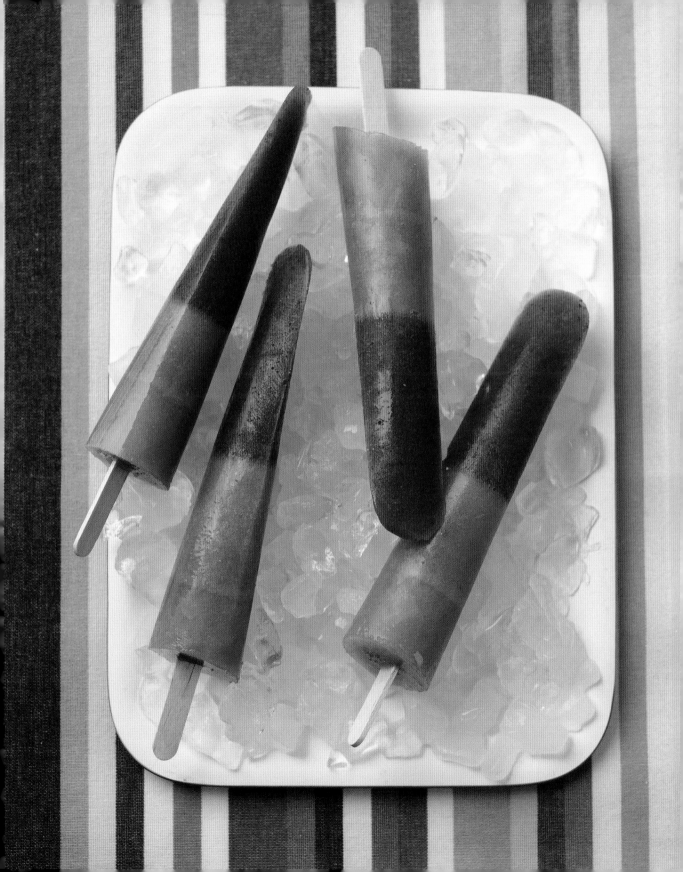

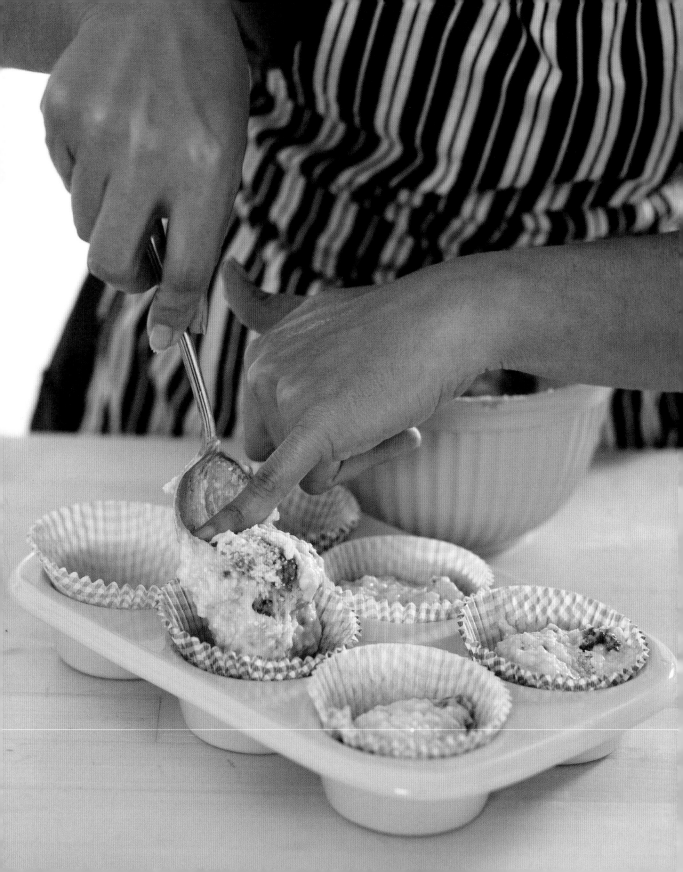

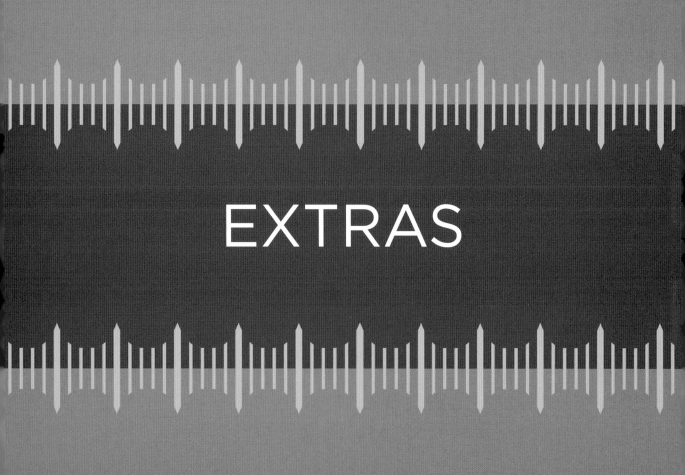

EXTRAS

Frostings

Homemade frosting is delicious and easy to make and can be used on cakes, cupcakes and brownies. Frosting is usually made from various combinations of high-fat ingredients such as milk, butter, cream cheese, whipped cream, soured cream and chocolate. People watching their fat intake can still enjoy frosted treats by using non-fat or low-fat frosting recipes. Buttercream frosting is a great multi-purpose frosting that works well with low-fat and non-fat substitutions. It can be made in a wide variety of flavours, and is easy to spread. It also works well for simple cake decorating needs.

Here's a collection of low-fat buttercream frosting recipes.

The method is the same for all these frostings. Simply put all the ingredients into a bowl and mix, using either a free-standing electric mixer or a hand whisk. An electric mixer gives a much better result because the sugar is properly incorporated into the low-fat spread and gives a lovely, creamy and velvety texture.

**ENOUGH FROSTING
FOR 12 SMALL CAKES
OR 1 LARGE CAKE**

1 Place all the frosting ingredients in a large heatproof bowl set over a pan of simmering water and stir until all the sugar is completely dissolved.

2 Now, using a hand-held electric mixer, whisk until thickened and soft peaks form.

3 Remove from the heat and continue to whisk until the mixture is cool.

4 Use a palette knife to spread the frosting over your cake or cakes.

Low-fat Zesty Lemon Buttercream

100g (3½oz) low-fat, heart-healthy spread
270g (10oz) icing sugar, sifted
grated zest of ½ lemon
1 tsp lemon essence
  (available in most large supermarkets.
  Stronger than lemon juice – and won't
  make the mixture runny!)
a little natural yellow food colouring

Low-fat Chocolate Frosting

100g (3½oz) low-fat, heart-healthy spread
270g (10oz) icing sugar, sifted
3 tbsp good-quality cocoa powder
skimmed milk if required

Low-fat Cream Cheese Frosting

450g (1lb) low-fat cream cheese
125g (4½oz) low-fat, heart-healthy spread
250g (9oz) icing sugar, sifted
1 tsp vanilla extract

Fat-free Italian Meringue Frosting

300g (10½oz) caster sugar
2 egg whites
1 tbsp lemon juice
3 tbsp orange juice

Low-fat Coconut Frosting

100g (3½oz) low-fat, heart-healthy spread
270g (10oz) icing sugar, sifted
90g (3oz) desiccated coconut

Virtually Fat-free Quark Frosting

Quark is a virtually fat-free soft cheese
that is readily available in supermarkets.
This frosting or cake filling has a slightly
sharper taste and goes wonderfully well
with both carrot cake and courgette
cake (see pages 24 and 34).

225g (8oz) Quark
  (virtually fat-free soft cheese)
2 tbsp lemon juice
20g (¾oz) icing sugar, sifted

Pomegranate Molasses

This is another delicious topping for any dessert. Pomegranates have very potent antioxidants that help keep us young, fight heart disease and prevent cancer. They are also a great source of vitamins B and C. This is delicious poured over ice cream, frozen yogurt or a scrummy cake.

**MAKES I LITRE
(1¾ PINTS)**

1 litre (1¾ pints)
   unsweetened
   pomegranate juice
115g (4oz) caster sugar
1 tbsp freshly squeezed
   lemon juice

TIP
Make sure the jar is perfectly clean beforehand by immersing in boiling water.

1 Add the pomegranate juice, sugar and lemon juice to a heavy-based saucepan and place over a medium heat.

2 Cook, stirring occasionally, until the sugar has completely dissolved. Once the sugar has dissolved, lower the heat to medium-low and cook until the mixture has reduced to 250ml (9fl oz). This will take about 1 hour. It should be the consistency of thick syrup.

3 Remove from the heat and allow to cool in the saucepan for 30 minutes. Transfer to a clean glass jar and allow to cool completely before covering and storing in the refrigerator for up to 6 months.

Raspberry Coulis

This coulis is a very simple addition to any dessert and it makes a lovely fresh sauce for ice cream, an accompaniment to cakes and also works well on top of pancakes. My daughter even likes a squirt on her porridge in the mornings!

**MAKES ABOUT
500ML (17FL OZ)**

250g (9oz) fresh or thawed
   raspberries
55g (2oz) granulated sugar
lemon juice to taste

1 Put the raspberries in a food processor or blender.

2 Heat the sugar and 5 tablespoons of water in a small pan over a medium heat until the sugar has dissolved, then bring to the boil for 2 minutes. Turn off the heat and let this mixture cool for 10 minutes before pouring over the raspberries.

3 Purée everything together in the food processor, then pass through a sieve to remove the seeds. Add a little lemon juice to taste. This should have a nice sharp tang to it! You can then use this straightaway or keep in the refrigerator for up to 2 weeks.

Quick & Easy Low-fat Creamy Custard

Making your own custard is great if you have time – but if you're a little pushed and want to give one of your desserts the perfect finishing touch, try this recipe. With health in mind, keep your portions sizes small but enjoy!

MAKES AROUND 8 SERVINGS

850ml (just under 1½ pints) low-fat instant custard in a carton
1 vanilla pod
150ml (5fl oz) low-fat crème fraîche

1 Put the low-fat custard in a bowl, then split the vanilla pod in half lengthways, scrape out the seeds with the tip of the knife and add the seeds to the custard.

2 Finally, using a hand whisk, whisk in the low-fat crème fraîche.

3 Transfer the custard to a pan and heat gently to the desired temperature, then serve.

Apple Sauce (Butter Replacement)

This is a simple recipe that can act as a replacement for butter in many recipes. So if you have a favourite recipe that uses butter, try to halve the amount, swap half for low-fat, heart-healthy spread and replace the other half with apple sauce. It works in some recipes and not in others, but give it a go and you might surprise yourself! I suggest you make double quantities of the apple sauce, as it will keep in the refrigerator for up to a week or in the freezer for up to three months.

1 To make apple purée, peel, core and slice cooking apples such as Bramley. You need 3–4 to make 470g (16½oz) of apple sauce. Place the apples in a pan with some water and cook gently until the apples are soft enough to mash to a pulp. This will take about 20 minutes. Keep adding water as you need it. You are aiming to have the apples soft and moist but not swimming in water.

2 Store in the refrigerator for up to a week or freeze in an ice-cube tray to use as needed for baking.

index

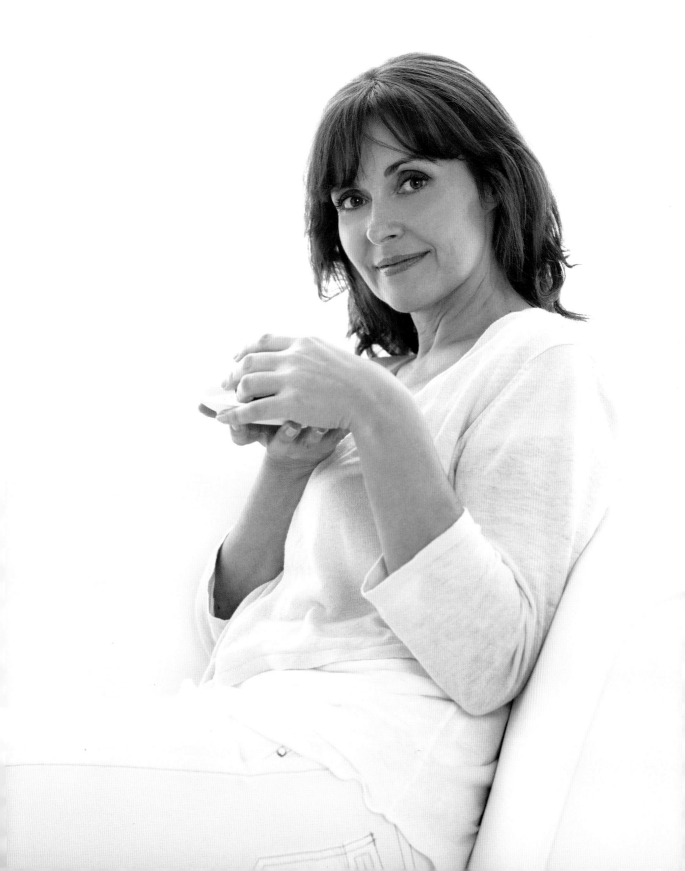

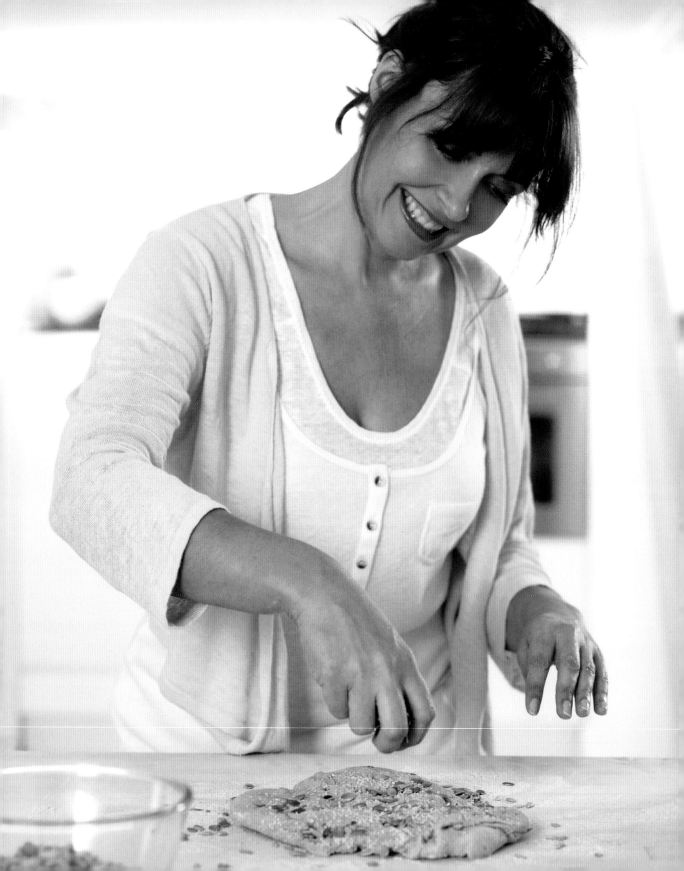